# 1 BASIC PRINCIPLES

## THE RADIOGRAPHIC IMAGE

The tissues that lie in the path of the X-ray beam absorb (i.e. attenuate) X-rays to differing degrees. These differences account for the radiographic image (Table 1.1 and Fig. 1.1).

**Table 1.1** Attenuation of the X-ray beam

| Tissue absorption | | Effect on the radiograph (see Fig. 1.1) |
|---|---|---|
| Least | Air or gas | Black image |
| | Fat | Dark grey image |
| | Soft tissue | Grey image |
| Most | Bone or calcium | White image |

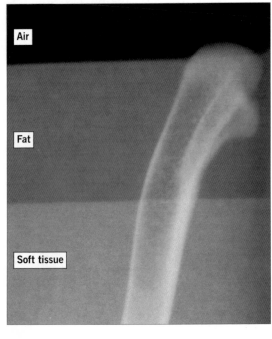

Air

Fat

Soft tissue

**Figure 1.1** *Tissues absorb the X-ray beam differently. Radiograph of a chicken leg (bone) partially submerged in a layer of vegetable oil (fat) floating on water (soft tissue). Note the difference in the blackening of the X-ray film.*

# ACCIDENT & EMERGENCY RADIOLOGY

## A SURVIVAL GUIDE

### SECOND EDITION

**Nigel Raby,** FRCR
Consultant Radiologist, Western Infirmary, Glasgow

**Laurence Berman,** FRCR
Consultant Radiologist, University Department of Radiology,
Addenbrooke's Hospital and University of Cambridge, Cambridge

**Gerald de Lacey,** FRCR
Consultant Radiologist, Northwick Park Hospital, London

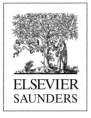

ELSEVIER
SAUNDERS

Philadelphia • Edinburgh • London • New York • Oxford • St Louis • Sydne

## ELSEVIER
### SAUNDERS

An imprint of Elsevier Ltd
© 2005 Elsevier Ltd. All rights reserved.

First edition © 1995 WB Saunders Company Ltd
Reprinted © 1999 Harcourt Publishers Ltd
Reprinted © 2002 Elsevier Science Ltd. All rights reserved
Reprinted © 2003 Elsevier Ltd. All rights reserved
Second edition © 2005 Elsevier Ltd. All rights reserved
Reprinted 2005

ISBN 0 7020 2667 0

**British Library Cataloguing in Publication Data**
A catalogue record for this book is available from the British Library

**Library of Congress Cataloging in Publication Data**
A catalog record for this book is available from the Library of Congress

**Notice**
Medical knowledge is constantly changing. Standard safety precautions must be followed, but as new research and clinical experience broaden our knowledge, changes in treatment and drug therapy may become necessary or appropriate. Readers are advised to check the most current product information provided by the manufacturer of each drug to be administered to verify the recommended dose, the method and duration of administration, and contraindications. It is the responsibility of the practitioner, relying on experience and knowledge of the patient, to determine dosages and the best treatment for each individual patient. Neither the Publisher nor the authors assume any liability for any injury and/or damage to persons or property arising from this publication.

**The Publisher**

Printed in Spain

print number : 9 8 7 6 5 4 3 2 1

tor: **Michael J Houston**
nt Manager: **Hilary Hewitt**
heryl Brant, Aoibhe O'Shea
apman
r: **Mick Ruddy**
nville

The Publisher's policy is to use paper manufactured from sustainable forests

Working together to grow libraries in developing countries
www.elsevier.com | www.bookaid.org | www.sabre.org

ELSEVIER   BOOK AID International   Sabre Foundation

# CONTENTS

# PREFACE

This is not a book of orthopaedic radiology . . . the purpose is to provide simple and systematic approaches to the evaluation of Emergency Department radiographs.

In this second edition we have aimed to make up for our original 1995 omissions, to remove inconsistencies, and to provide added value within each Chapter. The added value varies. In some chapters it represents additional radiological information, in others there are new explanatory drawings and/or improved radiographic illustrations. In some, it is simply an improvement in layout.

Changes have been substantial. For example, the chest radiograph is the most frequently requested radiological examination in the Emergency Department. Clearly a comprehensive description of thoracic abnormalities is not possible in a slip-into-my-pocket Survival Guide. All the same, over 90% of requests for a chest film are made in relation to ten clinical questions only. The chest chapter has been re-designed so as to address these specific queries. The skull chapter is another example. Skull radiography is now utilised much less frequently than in earlier years. Nevertheless, it is inevitable that paediatricians and Emergency Department doctors will request plain film radiography in some injured infants and children. Injudicious over-reading of a child's films may lead to consequences that are nearly as harmful as those resulting from under-reading. Radiographs may be interpreted as abnormal when a finding is simply due to an accessory suture. On other occasions a fracture may be erroneously interpreted as a normal suture or a developmental fissure. The skull chapter now includes a comprehensive set of illustrative drawings and radiographs which can assist with the accurate assessment and interpretation of an infant's or toddler's skull films.

The Key Points summary at the end of each chapter has been retained, but one feature is often highlighted on its own. The intention is to place an additional emphasis on a particularly subtle sign or appearance that is either not widely known or is regularly overlooked. Previously, references were kept to a minimum. They are now more extensive.

The Glossary acts as an additional chapter. We regard its enlargement as essential. Understanding the numerous terms used in radiological practice is important. We have added additional words and eponyms and have aimed to make all of the descriptions clear and unambiguous. Some recently introduced descriptive terms (such as the Madonna sign and the Scrapper's fracture) are now included. We have also included synonyms in order to overcome confusions in medical terminology that can occur between the United Kingdom and North America.

We have not attempted to provide a comprehensive text on all aspects of Emergency Department radiology. For example, several important abnormalities that are rarely missed – such as a Colles' fracture – have again been excluded.

Various statements will appear dogmatic, terse, and occasionally too oracular. This book is intended to help relatively inexperienced doctors who may have to make a radiological assessment at times when expert advice is not immediately available. As a consequence we have kept the caveats, exceptions, and qualifications to a minimum.

In each chapter we have assumed two important principles. Firstly, that clinical correlation with the radiographic findings must occur in each and every case. We take this as read. Secondly, that local guidelines indicating when to request plain film radiography will be applied. Guidelines and protocols vary from country to country and also between Emergency Departments within the same health care system. Accordingly, we have suggested relatively few when-to-request-radiology protocols.

Though this Survival Guide is designed primarily to assist doctors working in the Emergency Department it is hoped that it will be of value to others including radiologists, orthopaedic surgeons, and some paedatricians. The primary objective remains as before. To assist with answering the day in, day out, questions: these images look normal to me – but how can I be sure? Is there a subtle but important abnormality that I am overlooking?

Nigel Raby
Laurence Berman
Gerald de Lacey

November 2004

# ACKNOWLEDGEMENTS

In producing the first edition of the Survival Guide the authors were greatly indebted to Claire Gilman for her design and copy editing skills. Her high standards, patience, and hard work were invaluable. In this second edition others have made similarly important contributions. Dr Simon Morley at Northwick Park Hospital provided the new material to help with the assessment of skull films in infants and toddlers. His careful analysis of the embryology and radiographic anatomy in this difficult area was painstaking and yet another example of the student educating his teachers. The drawings in the first edition were provided by Dr Laurence Berman. For this second edition Nigel Webb, Medical Artist at Northwick Park and St. Mark's Hospitals, created additional illustrations. In order to ensure a coherent style Mick Ruddy of Elsevier arranged for the redrawing of all figures by Medical Artist Paul Banville. Mrs Pam Golden, at Northwick Park Hospital, typed draft after draft of the revisions and carried out the extensive secretarial tasks with a quiet efficiency. Without her crucial contribution this edition would not have been delivered on time. Our thanks are also due to Cheryl Brant of Elsevier for her invaluable help and patience with three demanding authors as she shepherded this Second Edition to completion.

Finally, two groups of doctors need to be acknowledged. They have had a profound influence on the drive to produce and now to improve this book. Firstly our teachers; those who taught us not only in the UK, but also in the USA, Canada and New Zealand. Just as importantly, we owe thanks to numerous stimulating and enthusiastic Registrars and Residents. We owe both of these groups a very great deal.

*A man can seldom – very, very, seldom fight a winning fight against his training: the odds are too heavy.*

Mark Twain

## FRACTURES

When a fracture results in separation of bone fragments, the X-ray beam that passes through the gap is not absorbed by bone. This results in a dark (lucent) line on the film. On the other hand, bone fragments may overlap or impact into each other. The resultant increased thickness of bone absorbs more of the X-ray beam and so results in a whiter (sclerotic or more dense) area on the film (Fig. 1.2).

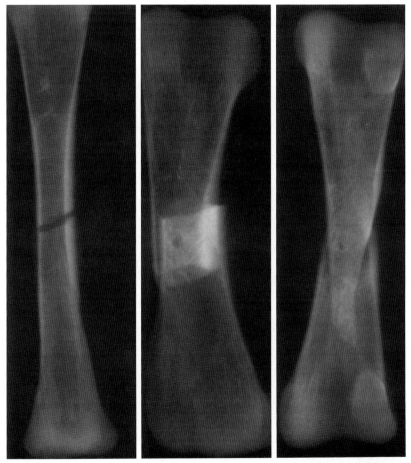

**Figure 1.2** *Three fractures. On the left the fragments are distracted and the fracture is identified by a dark black line on the radiograph. In the centre the fragments overlap and the fracture is identified by a dense region on the radiograph. On the right the fragments are impacted and produce an area of increased density.*

## THE PRINCIPLE OF TWO VIEWS

*'One view only is one view too few'*

■ Many fractures and dislocations are not detectable on a single view (Fig. 1.3). Consequently, it is normal practice to obtain two standard projections, usually at right angles to each other

■ Radiographic demonstration of a fracture usually depends on some separation or impaction of the fragments. This does not always occur and it is inevitable that some fractures will not be shown on the two standard views (Fig. 1.4). The principle of two views is in effect a compromise, albeit a practical one

■ At sites where fractures are known to be exceptionally difficult to detect (for example a suspected scaphoid fracture), it is routine practice to obtain more than two views.

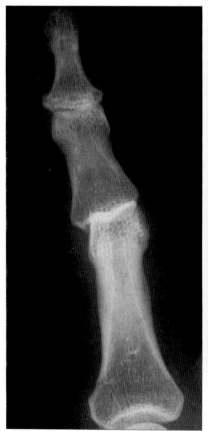
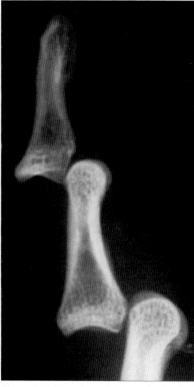

**Figure 1.3** *'One view only is one view too few'. Injured finger. The true extent of the injury is only evident from the lateral view.*

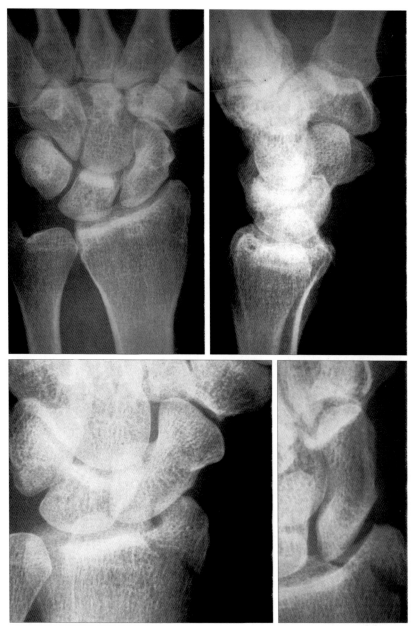

**Figure 1.4** *Fall on outstretched hand and injury to the distal radius. The standard PA and lateral views appear within normal limits. Two additional oblique views show an obvious fracture involving the styloid process of the radius. The normal practice of obtaining two views is a compromise. It is inevitable that the standard projections will sometimes fail to show an undisplaced fracture.*

## INDIRECT EVIDENCE OF A FRACTURE

There are radiological soft tissue signs which can provide a clue that a fracture is likely. These include displacement of the elbow fat pads (pages 93, 96) or the presence of a fluid level (Knee, page 206; Skull, page 26).

## PATIENT POSITION AND DIRECTION OF THE X-RAY BEAM

■ Knowledge of the patient's position during radiography is important. The radiograph may have been obtained with the patient supine or erect (Figs 1.5, 1.6)

■ A fluid level will only be shown when a radiograph is obtained using a horizontal X-ray beam (i.e. the beam is parallel to the floor). A vertical beam radiograph (i.e. the X-ray beam is at right angles to the floor) will not reveal a fluid level.

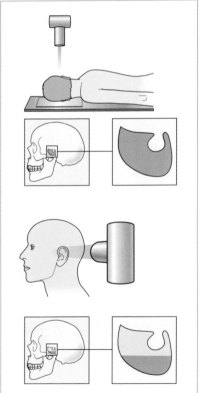

**Figure 1.5** *Blood in the sphenoid sinus. A fluid level can only be demonstrated when a horizontal X-ray beam is used.*

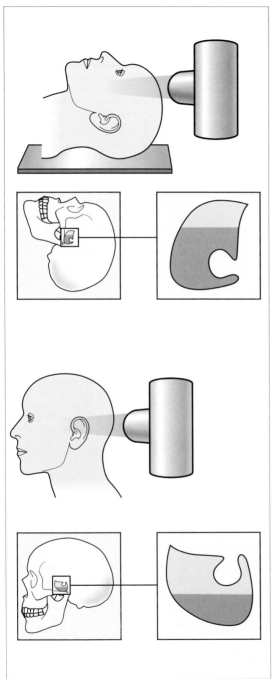

**Figure 1.6** *Blood in the sphenoid sinus. Radiographs obtained with a horizontal beam. The orientation of a fluid level depends on the position of the patient.*

## DESCRIBING A FRACTURE

- The radiographic appearance needs to be described in a consistent style using accepted terminology (Tables 1.2 and 1.3)
- Fractures that are particular to children are described on pages 306–315.

---

**Table 1.2** A fracture involving a long bone[1,2]

**GENERAL**

*Site*
The shaft of a long bone
is divided into thirds:
- Proximal
- Middle
- Distal

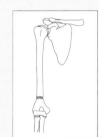

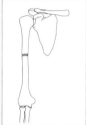

**Fracture of**
**distal third**

**Fracture at junction of**
**proximal and middle thirds**

*Fracture line*

- Transverse. At right
  angles to the long axis
  of the bone
- Oblique. At an angle of
  less than 90° to the
  long axis of the bone
- Spiral. Curving and
  twisting along the bone

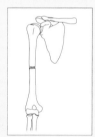

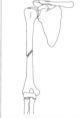

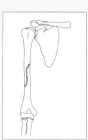

**Transverse**

**Oblique**

**Spiral**

*Comminution*
More than two fragments

*Impaction*
One fragment is driven
into the other

*Intra-articular*
Involvement of an
articular surface

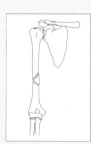

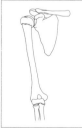

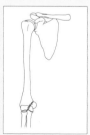

**Comminuted**

**Impacted**

**Intra-articular**

**Table 1.2** Continued

**POSITION**

*Deformity*
- None
- Displacement: i.e. the bone ends have shifted relative to each other – the direction of displacement is described with reference to *the position of the distal fragment*

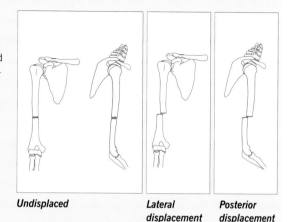

| **Undisplaced** | **Lateral displacement** | **Posterior displacement** |

*Angulation*

May be described *either* by reference to the direction in which the apex of the fracture points *or* by indicating the direction of tilt of the distal fragment. *To avoid confusion, the latter convention is recommended*

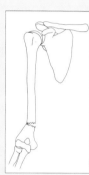 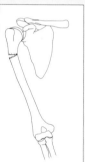 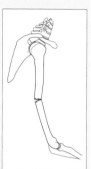

| **Lateral tilt of the distal fragment** | **Medial tilt of the distal fragment** | **Anterior tilt of the distal fragment** |

**ROTATION**
See Chapter 20, page 333

1. Pitt MJ, Speer DP. Radiologic reporting of skeletal trauma. Radiol Clin North Am 1990; 28: 247–256.
2. Renner RR, Mauler GG, Ambrose JL. The radiologist, the orthopedist, the lawyer, and the fracture. Semin Roentgenol 1978; 13: 7–18.

**Table 1.3** Subluxation and dislocation

| NORMAL | SUBLUXATION | DISLOCATION |
|---|---|---|
| | The articular surface of one bone maintains some contact with the articular surface of the adjacent bone. The joint surfaces are no longer congruous but contact has not been completely disrupted | The articular surfaces at the joint have lost all contact with each other. There is complete disarticulation |

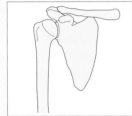 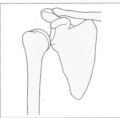 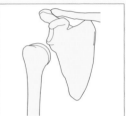

## SOME NORMAL APPEARANCES CAN SIMULATE FRACTURES[3]

The most important consideration in deciding whether a particular radiographic finding is significant is correlation with the clinical examination. Frequently, it is necessary to re-examine the patient to look for swelling or tenderness at a specific site in order to properly assess the relevance of a particular radiographic appearance.

### VASCULAR MARKINGS

A nutrient vessel may result in a dark (lucent) line in the cortex of a long bone (Fig. 1.7). This line may mimic a fracture. When seen in profile the line runs obliquely through one cortex only, from the inner to the outer margin. When seen *en face* at least one of the margins will appear sclerotic (dense).

### ACCESSORY OSSICLES

These small bones can mimic fracture fragments. They are particularly common around the foot and ankle.

■ An ossicle has a well defined sclerotic (white) margin (Fig. 1.8). The bones adjacent to the ossicle are normal

■ A recent fracture fragment will have at least one edge where the sclerotic margin is either absent (Fig. 1.9) or irregular. Often, one of the adjacent bones will show a similar irregular margin indicating the site of origin of the fragment.

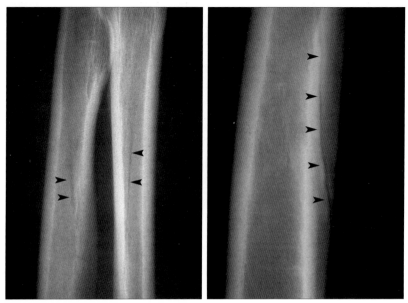

**Figure 1.7** *Pitfall. Nutrient grooves in long bones may produce an appearance that mimics a fracture. The clinical examination will usually indicate whether the finding is due to a fracture or to a groove.*

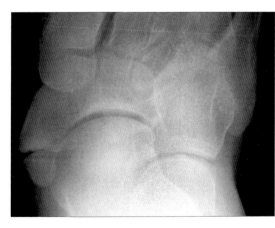

**Figure 1.8** *Normal accessory ossicles need to be distinguished from fracture fragments. This accessory ossicle (an os tibiale externum) has a well-defined margin and the adjacent bones are normal.*

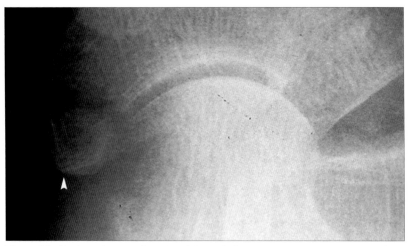

**Figure 1.9** *The bone fragment (arrowhead) has a similar appearance to the accessory ossicle in Figure 1.8, but the cortex is irregular and poorly defined. The adjacent bone is also abnormal. This is a fracture of the navicular.*

## EPIPHYSES AND GROWTH PLATES

Sometimes a growth plate may be mistaken for a fracture. Distinguishing between normal and abnormal can be difficult (Fig. 1.10). When there is uncertainty it is best to seek expert advice. Also, Keats' *Atlas*[3] will be helpful.

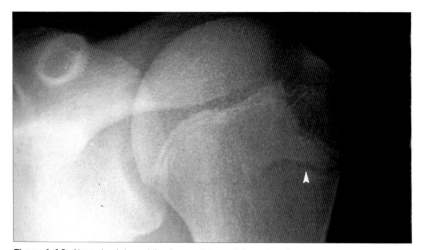

**Figure 1.10** *Normal epiphyseal line in an adolescent (arrowhead).*

3. Keats TE. Atlas of normal roentgen variants that may simulate disease, 7th ed. Year Book Medical Publishers, Chicago, 2001.

## KNOWLEDGE OF NORMAL ANATOMY

The accurate interpretation of most radiographic images depends in large part on a sound understanding of basic skeletal anatomy. To test your knowledge, cover the captions and name the numbered bones and/or structures on the next three pages.

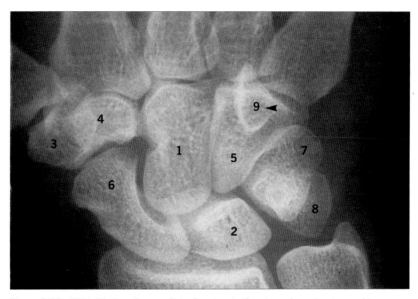

**Figure 1.11** *Wrist. PA view. 1 = capitate; 2 = lunate; 3 = trapezium; 4 = trapezoid; 5 = hamate; 6 = scaphoid; 7 = triquetral; 8 = pisiform; 9 = hook of the hamate.*

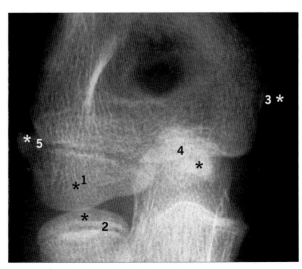

**Figure 1.12** *Normal paediatric elbow. AP view. The asterisks mark the epiphyses: 1 = capitellum; 2 = head of radius; 3 = medial (or internal) epicondyle; 4 = trochlear; 5 = lateral (or external) epicondyle.*

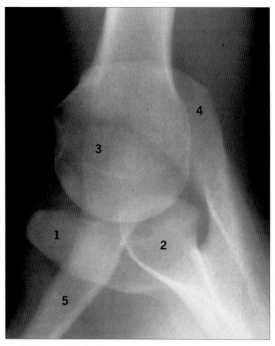

**Figure 1.13** *Shoulder. Axial view. 1 = coracoid process of the scapula; 2 = glenoid; 3 = lateral end of the clavicle; 4 = acromion; 5 = clavicle.*

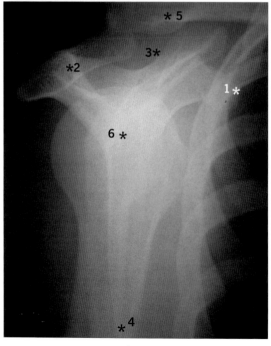

**Figure 1.14** *Shoulder. The 'Y' view. 1 = coracoid process of scapula; 2 = acromion; 3 = superior margin of blade of the scapula; 4 = blade of scapula; 5 = clavicle; 6 = head of humerus projected over the centre of the glenoid.*

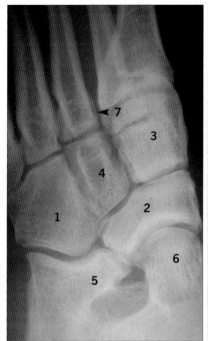

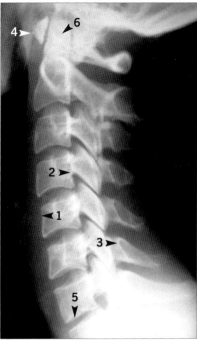

**Figure 1.15** *Foot. Oblique view. 1 = cuboid; 2 = navicular; 3 = medial and intermediate cuneiforms superimposed over each other; 4 = lateral cuneiform; 5 = calcaneum; 6 = talus; 7 = medial margin of the base of the third metatarsal.*

**Figure 1.16** *Cervical spine. Lateral view. 1 = anterior margin of C5; 2 = pedicle of C4; 3 = base of the spinous process of C6 (or posterior margin of the spinal canal); 4 = anterior arch of C1; 5 = inferior end plate of C7 vertebral body; 6 = odontoid peg.*

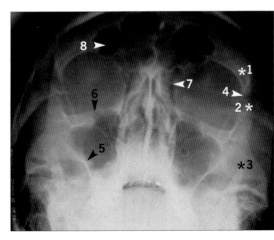

**Figure 1.17** *Face. OM view. 1 = zygomatic process of the frontal bone; 2 = frontal process of the zygomatic bone; 3 = zygoma; 4 = synchondrosis (suture) between 1 and 2; 5 = lateral wall of the maxillary antrum; 6 = inferior orbital margin; 7 = ethmoid sinus; 8 = frontal sinus.*

# 2 SKULL

- Following an apparently mild head injury there should be few requests for skull radiography (SXR).[1–4] The compelling evidence is based on a meta-analysis of 20 head injury surveys[3]

- Advocates for the minimal use of SXR do not propose that all mild head injury patients should be referred for CT instead.[2] *It remains a point of principle that CT is only indicated in a patient whose clinical condition raises a reasonable concern that a treatable intracranial haemorrhage might be present*

- Evaluating a SXR in infants and very young children following trauma presents unique problems. Misinterpreting a suture as a fracture, or a fracture as an accessory suture, may have serious consequences. A basic understanding of the locations and general appearance of these sutures will help to reduce the likelihood of misdiagnosis.

## BASIC RADIOGRAPHS

Two projections are standard practice.

- **Lateral.** Obtained with a horizontal X-ray beam (Figs 2.1, 2.2)

- **One additional view.** The projection will depend on the site of injury. Trauma to the occipital bone requires a Towne's view (Figs 2.3, 2.4). For any other injury an AP frontal view is required (Fig. 2.5). Obtaining both a Towne's and an AP frontal view is unnecessary.[5]

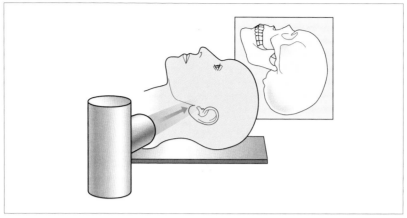

**Figure 2.1** *Lateral view. The patient is lying down. The importance of patient position and the use of a horizontal X-ray beam is described in Chapter 1 (page 6).*

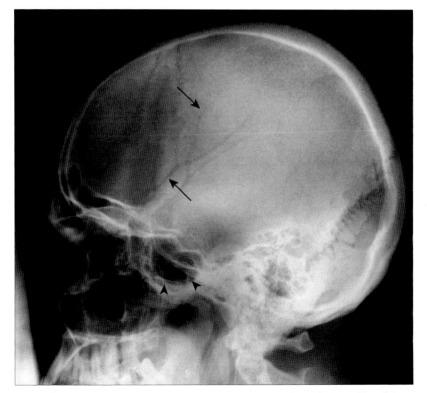

**Figure 2.2** *Normal lateral view. Note: typical vascular markings (arrows); the position of the sphenoid sinus (arrowheads).*

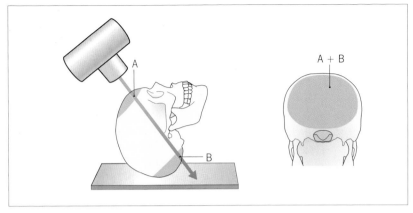

**Figure 2.3** *Towne's view. This radiograph is obtained primarily to show the occipital bone. Note that the frontal and occipital bones are superimposed. As a consequence, a fracture through the frontal bone may also be visualised on this radiograph.*

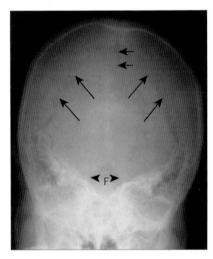

**Figure 2.4** *Normal Towne's view. The sagittal suture (arrowheads), the lambdoid suture (large arrows) and the margin (arrowheads) of the foramen magnum (F).*

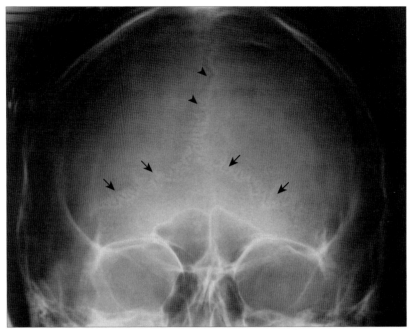

**Figure 2.5** *The skull vault as shown on the normal AP frontal radiograph. Note the foreshortened sagittal suture (arrowheads) and the lambdoid suture (arrows).*

## ANATOMY

Most difficulties arise because a normal appearance can be mistaken for an abnormality. These false positive diagnoses can be reduced by being familiar with:

■ **The normal sutures and accessory sutures.** Specifically the position and appearance of:

❏ the three large sutures: the lambdoid, coronal and sagittal (Figs 2.4 and 2.5)

❏ the other smaller sutures around the mastoid bones

❏ the common accessory sutures found in some infants and young children – see *Infants and toddlers* (pp. 28–43)

■ **The metopic suture.** This is the most common accessory suture persisting in adults (Fig. 2.6)

■ **Vascular impressions.** Specifically:

❏ the sites of the most common vessel grooves/markings (Fig. 2.2)

❏ the radiographic features that help to distinguish between a fracture and a **vessel** marking (Table 2.1)

■ **The normal sphenoid sinus**

❏ in young children it is not pneumatised

❏ in adults it contains air; the amount of pneumatisation causes the radiographic appearance to vary widely between individuals (Fig. 2.7).

**Table 2.1** Distinguishing features

| Vascular marking | Fracture |
|---|---|
| Appears grey, because the vessel lies in a groove and consequently only the inner table of the skull is thinned (Fig. 2.8) | Frequently appears black, because the inner and outer skull tables are breached |
| Has branches that gradually decrease in size as the vessel extends peripherally | Has branches that do not taper (i.e. do not decrease in size) in a uniform manner |
| Has well-defined white (sclerotic) margins | Does not have a well-defined white (sclerotic) margin |

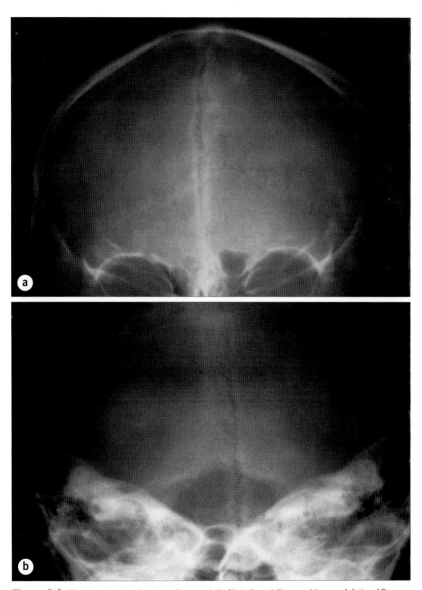

**Figure 2.6** *Persistent metopic suture in an adult. Note its midline position on **(a)** the AP frontal radiograph and on **(b)** the Towne's view where it crosses the foramen magnum.*

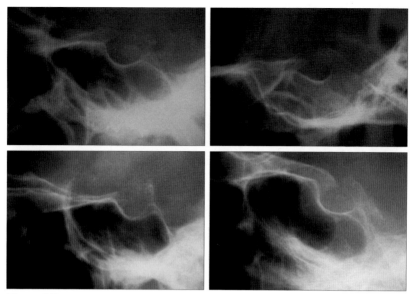

**Figure 2.7** *Variable appearance of the normal sphenoid sinus. Variation occurs in older children and adults because of individual differences in pneumatisation.*

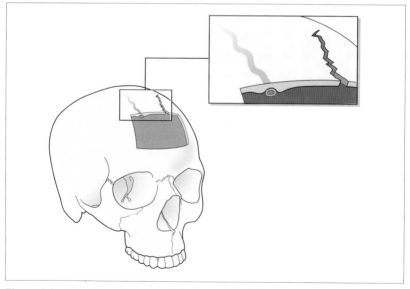

**Figure 2.8** *A blood vessel grooves only the inner table of the skull. The resultant marking appears as a grey line on the radiograph. A fracture involves the full thickness of the skull; as a consequence the fracture appears as a very black line.*

## INJURIES – ADULTS AND OLDER CHILDREN

In practice, the detection of an abnormality is easy. There are only four features that indicate that a fracture is present, and one of these is very rare. The radiographs need to be checked/inspected in a systematic manner.

## SYSTEMATIC INSPECTION OF THE SXR: 3 STEPS

### Step 1
Scrutinise the area on the radiograph which corresponds to the site of injury. Use a bright light – or vary the windowing – if necessary.

### Step 2
Look for three important abnormalities:

- *Linear fracture.* A lucent (black) line (Figs 2.9, 2.10)

- *Depressed fracture.* A dense white area or parallel white lines due to overlapping or rotated bone fragments (Figs 2.11, 2.12)

- *Fluid level in the sphenoid sinus.* This will be visible on the lateral film since the radiograph is taken using a horizontal X-ray beam. A fluid level:

  - indicates haemorrhage or CSF within the sinus and suggests that a base of skull fracture is present (Figs 2.13–2.15)

  - may be the only abnormality on the radiograph. Detection of a fluid level will affect management since a fracture involving the sphenoid sinus is a compound fracture.

### Step 3
Look for one exceptionally rare abnormality:

- *Intracranial air.* Seen as lucent (black) areas in any of several positions: in the frontal region, in a basal cistern, between cerebral sulci or in a lateral ventricle (Fig. 2.16). In the context of a seemingly mild head injury the presence of intracranial air indicates that a fracture involves either a frontal sinus or the sphenoid sinus.

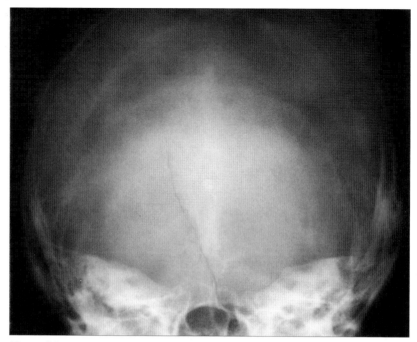

**Figure 2.9** *Towne's view. A linear fracture through the occipital bone.*

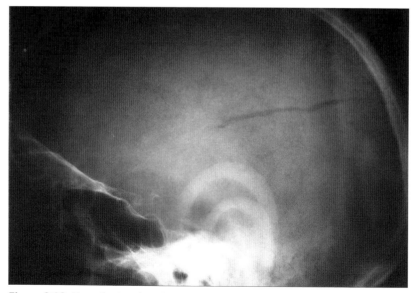

**Figure 2.10** *Linear fracture through the parietal bone.*

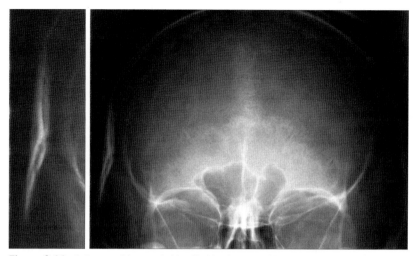

**Figure 2.11** *A depressed fracture is identified by the area of increased density (i.e. sclerotic/whiter).*

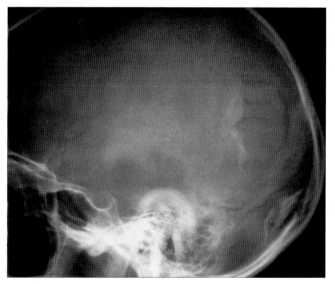

**Figure 2.12** *Extensive parieto-occipital fracture with both linear (black) and depressed (white) components.*

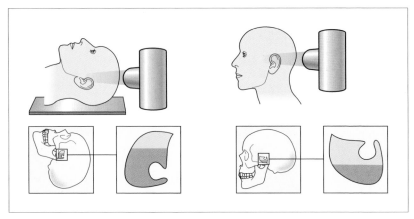

**Figure 2.13** *The appearance of a fluid level in the sphenoid sinus will depend on the position of the patient. It is important to know how the patient's lateral view has been obtained.*

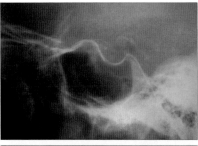 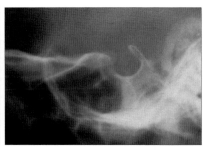

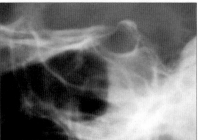

**Figure 2.14** *Fluid level in the sphenoid sinus in three different patients. A fluid level indicates a fracture through the base of the skull. Each radiograph was obtained with the patient supine and using a horizontal X-ray beam.*

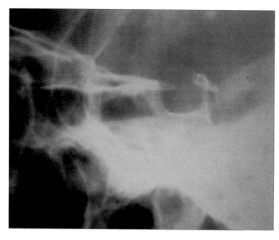

**Figure 2.15** *A fluid level in the sphenoid sinus is the only radiographic evidence of a basal skull fracture in this patient. This radiograph was obtained with the patient sitting up.*

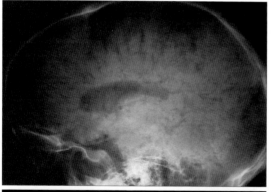

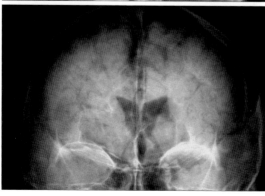

**Figure 2.16** *Intracranial air resulting from a fracture that involved a sinus. Air is present in the cerebral sulci, the lateral ventricles and the basal cisterns.*

## INJURIES – INFANTS AND TODDLERS

The assessment of the SXR of a neonate, infant or young child (toddler) requires a meticulous step-by-step approach.[6,7] The clinical concern is the need not to overlook nor to incorrectly diagnose a non-accidental injury (NAI).

---

**Table 2.2** A basic classification of skull sutures in infants and toddlers

A. **The normal sutures:**

*Visible on the SXR in all infants and toddlers – persisting in all adults*

Sagittal

Coronal

Lambdoid

Squamosal

Smaller sutures around the mastoid

B. **A normal developmental suture:**

*Visible on the SXR in all infants and many toddlers – but not in adults*

Innominate

C. **The most common accessory sutures:**

*Visible on the SXR in some infants and toddlers – very occasionally persisting in a few adults*

Metopic

Accessory parietal

Mendosal

---

## THE QUESTION: IS IT A SUTURE OR IS IT A FRACTURE?

### ■ General principles 1

■ Wide sutures are normal in neonates

■ A normal skull suture, an accessory suture or a wormian bone (see page 336) can mimic a fracture.[8–12]

■ Accessory sutures are common and are a part of normal development

■ An awareness of the positions and appearances of the common accessory sutures can help to reduce errors of interpretation.

■ Radiography in infants can be very difficult. The Towne's view (injury to occiput) or the AP frontal view (injury elsewhere) is frequently a technical compromise. The head is often slightly rotated.

### ■ General principles 2

■ The age at which an accessory suture closes is variable

■ Accessory sutures are present in some older children – very occasionally they persist into adulthood (Fig. 2.6). The positions of the normal sutures and of the more common accessory sutures (Table 2.2) are shown in Figs 2.17–2.35

■ Various authors use different descriptive terms/names (Table 2.3).

**Table 2.3** Synonyms

| Term | Also known as |
| --- | --- |
| Incomplete suture | Fissure |
| Accessory parietal suture | Intraparietal suture |
| Mendosal suture | Transverse occipital suture |
| Innominate suture | Innominate synchondrosis |

## A PRACTICAL APPROACH TO ASSESSING AN INFANT'S OR TODDLER'S SXR

### FIRST
#### Examine the site of injury

Look for evidence of a fracture using Step **1** and the first two parts of Step **2** as for adults and older children (page 23).

### SECOND
#### Assess the frontal projection (Fig. 2.17)

■ Trace the lambdoid suture

❑ It is common to see one (or several) wormian bones. This is a normal finding. A wormian bone is a small area of the skull (sometimes as large as 1–2 cm in diameter) within a suture. The bone is completely surrounded by the suture (Figs 2.17, 2.18)

❑ The lambdoid suture meets the sagittal suture in the midline. On the frontal radiograph the sagittal suture appears foreshortened

■ Trace the sagittal suture

❑ Where it meets the coronal suture, the sagittal suture should stop. If it continues below this point then the patient has a metopic suture. This accessory suture divides the frontal bone into two halves (Figs 2.19, 2.20). The metopic suture is the commonest accessory suture in children. Sometimes it persists into adulthood

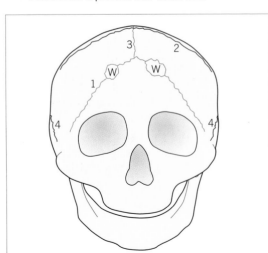

**Figure 2.17** *Normal sutures on the frontal view. This diagram also shows two wormian bones contained within the lambdoid suture.*
*1 = lambdoid suture;*
*2 = coronal suture;*
*3 = sagittal suture;*
*4 = squamosal suture;*
*W = wormian bone.*
*(Note: The following Figures 2.18, 2.21, 2.25 derive from this numbering convention.)*

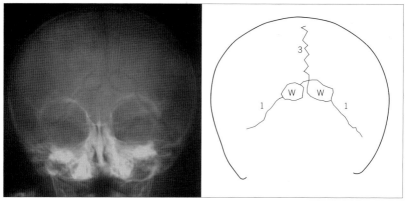

**Figure 2.18** *Normal sutures, present in all children. Frontal view (fronto-occipital).*
*This lambdoid suture contains two wormian bones. 1 = lambdoid suture; 3 = sagittal suture.*

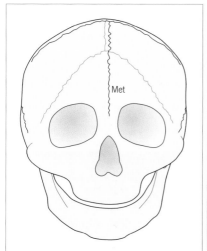

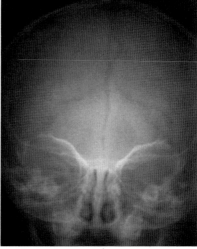

**Figure 2.19** *Accessory suture –*
*the metopic (Met). It divides the frontal*
*bone into two halves.*

**Figure 2.20** *Accessory suture – the metopic.*
*Incidentally, a wormian bone is present in the*
*sagittal suture and another lies within the*
*lambdoid suture. Wormian bones are*
*commonplace.*

■ Examine the parietal bone

❏ Is an accessory parietal suture present? Accessory parietal sutures are not exceptional. Of all the accessory sutures these are the ones that cause the most confusion

❏ Accessory parietal sutures may be complete or incomplete (Figs 2.21, 2.22, 2.31). They may be present on the frontal projection.

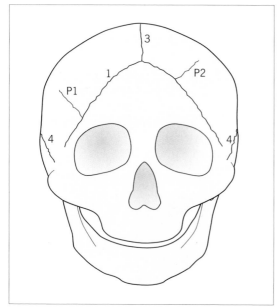

**Figure 2.21** *Possible positions/sites of accessory parietal sutures.*
*1 = lambdoid suture;*
*3 = sagittal suture;*
*4 = squamosal suture;*
*P1 = accessory parietal suture;*
*P2 = accessory parietal suture.*

**Figure 2.22** *Accessory parietal suture (arrow).*

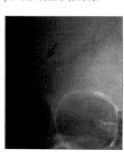

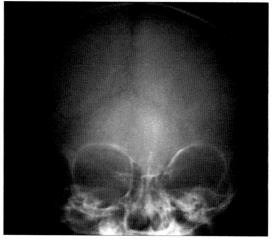

## Assess the Towne's projection (Fig. 2.23)

■ Examine the occipital bone. Trace the normal sutures (Fig. 2.24). Accessory sutures may be present.

  ❑ **the mendosal suture**. It may be present on both sides. It can be complete or incomplete; most commonly incomplete (Figs 2.25, 2.26)

  ❑ **midline and lateral incomplete sutures**. These accessory sutures are very rare. They extend from the posterior margin of the foramen magnum for a length of 1–2 cm. When present they are usually only visible on a technically good Towne's view.

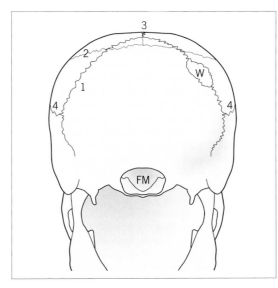

**Figure 2.23** *Normal sutures on the Towne's view. A wormian bone is shown. 1 = lambdoid suture; 2 = coronal suture; 3 = sagittal suture; 4 = squamosal suture; W = wormian bone; FM = foramen magnum.*

**Figure 2.24** *(Below) Normal sutures present in all children. Towne's view. 1 = lambdoid suture; 2 = coronal suture; 3 = sagittal suture.*

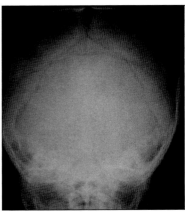
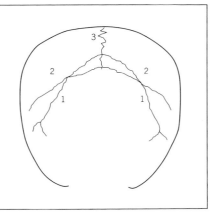

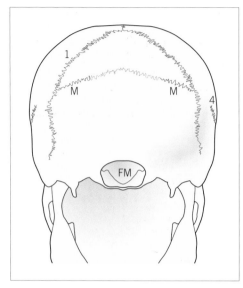

**Figure 2.25** *Accessory suture – the mendosal (M). It is situated in the occipital bone. Very occasionally it is whole (i.e. complete). More often it is incomplete. Very often it is incomplete and on one side of the bone only.*
*1 = lambdoid suture;*
*4 = squamosal suture;*
*FM = foramen magnum.*

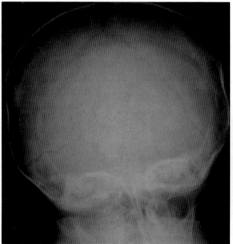
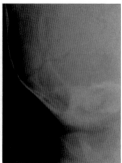

**Figure 2.26** *Accessory suture – the mendosal. It may be whole (i.e. complete). Usually it is incomplete. In this patient it is incomplete and on one side of the occipital bone only.*

**Pitfall** The appearance of a normal squamosal suture on the Towne's or frontal radiograph may confuse the unwary. Because it is situated on the side of the skull it is seen tangentially and can mimic a lucent fracture line. An incorrect diagnosis of a fracture is most likely to occur when the two squamosal sutures are developmentally asymmetrical and/or the patient is slightly rotated (Fig. 2.27).

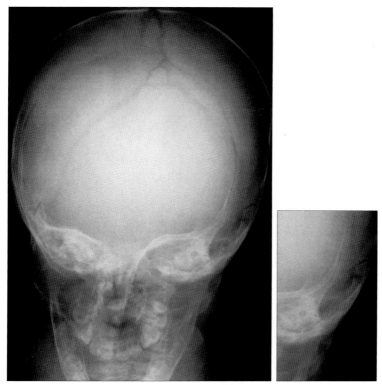

**Figure 2.27** *Pitfall. A normal squamosal suture can appear unduly prominent and may be mistaken for a fracture. The usual cause for asymmetry and/or a prominent appearance is patient rotation on a Towne's or frontal projection. The very prominent left squamosal suture in this patient is caused by slight rotation of the head.*

## THIRD
### Assess the lateral projection (Fig. 2.28)

■ The sagittal suture is not seen on this radiograph because the suture lies in the midline parallel to the film. For the same reason a metopic suture will not be detected on the lateral radiograph

■ If the patient is very slightly rotated, then the two halves of the coronal suture can appear as two parallel lines (Fig. 2.29). The same applies to the two halves of the lambdoid suture

■ Accessory parietal sutures are often best seen on this view (Figs 2.31, 2.33)

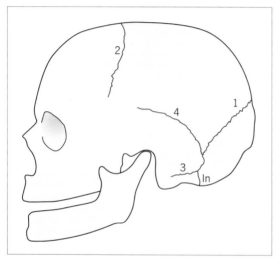

**Figure 2.28** *Normal sutures. The common normal sutures, present in all infants and toddlers and seen on most lateral SXRs.*
*1 = lambdoid suture;*
*2 = coronal suture;*
*3 = occipitomastoid suture;*
*4 = squamosal suture;*
*In = innominate suture.*

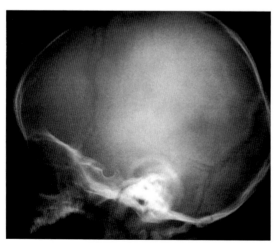

**Figure 2.29** *Normal sutures.* **Note:** *slight rotation of the patient may cause some of these sutures to appear as double lines or to be projected high or low on the radiograph. Rotation causes the two sides of the coronal suture to be seen in this patient.*

## The lateral projection (continued)

■ Trace the lambdoid suture. As it nears the base of the skull (in the region of the mastoid bone) the suture seems to be complex (Figs 2.29, 2.33). This seemingly tangled appearance is mainly caused by overlapping of the normal occipitomastoid sutures on the right and left sides. Don't worry about this. However, posterior to this complex and arising from the lambdoid suture there will be a normal suture, and a normal developmental suture. Occasionally there will also be an accessory suture

❑ *The normal suture* is the **squamosal suture**. It extends anteriorly, separating the parietal bone from the temporal bone. The usual appearance is of a pair of lines on the lateral projection (i.e. the left squamosal suture and the right squamosal suture). Invariably, the squamosal suture fades away as it passes anteriorly (Fig. 2.28)

❑ *The normal developmental suture* is the **innominate suture** (Figs 2.28, 2.29). It is present in all neonates. It rarely persists in adults. This suture is situated posterior to the normal occipitomastoid suture

❑ *The accessory suture* is **the mendosal suture**. It extends posteriorly (Figs 2.30, 2.34, 2.35).

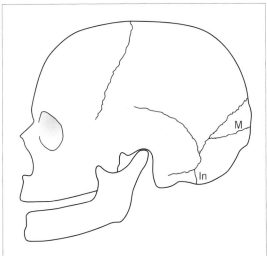

**Figure 2.30** *To show the position of the innominate suture (In) and the mendosal suture (M).*

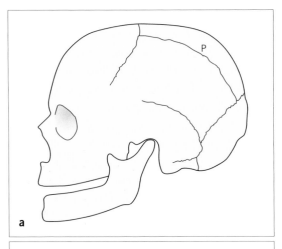

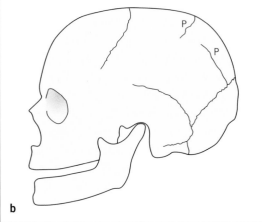

**Figure 2.31** *Diagrammatic representation of three different accessory parietal (P) sutures. (a) A complete suture; horizontal. (b) Two incomplete sutures. One is horizontal, the other is vertical.*

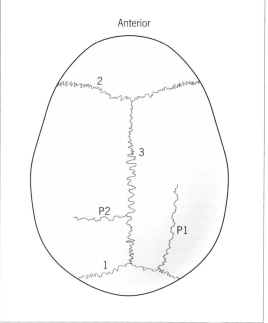

**Figure 2.32** *Accessory parietal sutures vary in position. This drawing does not correspond to any radiographic projection. It shows the general positions and direction of the more common incomplete accessory parietal sutures (P1 and P2) when looking down from above at the cranium. 1 = lambdoid suture; 2 = coronal suture; 3 = sagittal suture.*

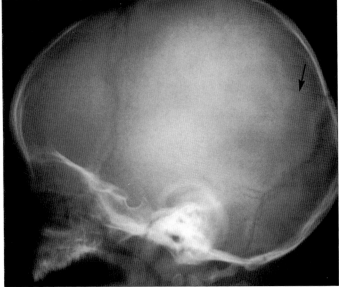

**Figure 2.33** *An incomplete accessory parietal suture situated just above the lambdoid suture.*

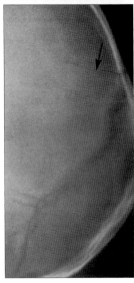

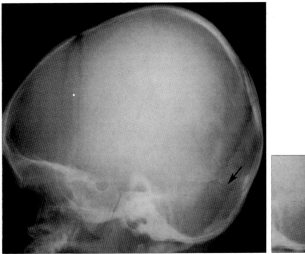
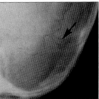

**Figure 2.34** *Two incomplete mendosal sutures extend posteriorly and horizontally from the lambdoid suture. Of course, these two mendosal sutures do not arise on the same side of the skull; one incomplete suture is on the left side of the occipital bone, the other is on the right side.*

*Incidentally, note the lucent line that represents the spheno-occipital synchondrosis, situated at the base of the skull inferior and posterior to the pituitary fossa. It is not a fracture. This unossified line is a normal appearance in all infants. This synchondrosis is also present in Figure 2.33.*

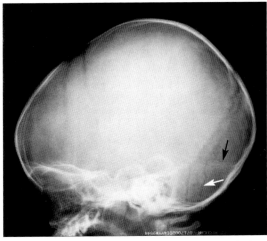
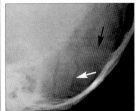

**Figure 2.35** *Incomplete mendosal sutures extending horizontally (black arrow).*
**Note:** *the innominate suture (present in all infants) is also seen on both sides (white arrow).*

## FOURTH

### Always apply three cardinal principles.

■ Whenever a lucent line is detected on an infant's or a child's SXR it is essential to examine the two radiographs together (Fig. 2.36). They form a complementary pair

■ The radiological findings must always be correlated with the clinical history and the physical examination.

■ Be very careful in rushing too swiftly to judgement. Observing an abnormality is important. Circumspection, and an informed approach, is then required when assigning a particular significance to the abnormality[13–21]

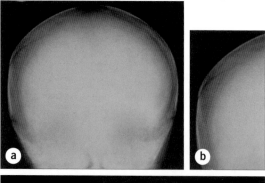

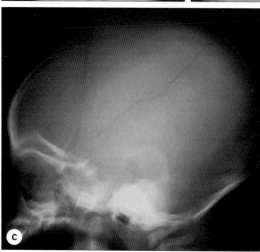

**Figure 2.36** *It is important that the two SXR views are evaluated as a pair. They complement each other. On the frontal SXR (a, b) the lucent line could be interpreted as an accessory parietal suture. The lateral view (c) shows that the line is much more extensive and continues through to involve the temporal bone. This is a fracture.*

**Table 2.4** Summary notes on accessory sutures

| | Most commonly seen on these radiographs | | Notes |
|---|---|---|---|
| **Metopic suture** | Frontal | ✓✓ | The commonest accessory suture that persists in older children and adults |
| | Towne's | ✓ | |
| **Accessory parietal suture** | Towne's | ✓✓ | May be complete or incomplete. Occur in vertical, horizontal or oblique orientations. Most commonly vertical |
| | Frontal | ✓ | |
| | Lateral | ✓ | |
| **Mendosal suture** | Lateral | ✓✓ | Extends posteriorly from the lambdoid suture on the lateral view. Passes medially on the Towne's view |
| | Towne's | ✓ | |
| **Innominate suture** | Lateral | ✓✓ | Sometimes classified as an accessory suture but best regarded/classified as a normal developmental suture because *it is always present* in infants. As the child matures the suture disappears |

## KEY POINTS 1

Skull fractures in adults – look for

■ Three abnormalities

❏ linear fracture = lucent line (black on radiograph)

❏ depressed fracture = dense line (white on radiograph)

❏ fluid level in the sphenoid sinus = base of skull fracture

■ One very rare abnormality

❏ intracranial air = a fracture involving a sinus

## KEY POINTS 2

Skull fractures in infants and toddlers – remember

■ Accessory sutures are common

■ Calling an accessory suture a fracture may lead to an incorrect suggestion of NAI

■ Dismissing a fracture as an accessory suture can have serious clinical consequences

■ To avoid mistakes:

❏ be aware of the positions of the most common accessory sutures

❏ assess and interpret an infant's or toddler's radiographs in a systematic step-by-step manner

# REFERENCES

1. Hackney DB. Skull radiography in the evaluation of trauma: a survey of current practice. Radiology 1991; 181: 711–714.
2. Moseley I. Skull fractures and mild head injury. J Neurol Neurosurg Psychiatry 2000; 68: 403–404.
3. Hofman PAM, Nelemans P, Kemerink GJ et al. Value of radiological diagnosis of skull fracture in the management of mild head injury: meta-analysis. J Neurol Neurosurg Psychiatry 2000: 68: 416–422.
4. Frush DP, O'Hara SM, Kliewer MA. Pediatric imaging perspective: acute head trauma – is skull radiography useful? J Pediatrics 1998; 132: 553–554.
5. McGlinchey I, Fleet MF, Eatock FC, Raby ND. A comparison of two or three radiographic views in the diagnosis of skull fractures. Clin Radiol 1998; 53: 215–217.
6. Mogbo KI, Slovis TL, Canady AI et al. Appropriate imaging in children with skull fractures and suspicion of abuse. Radiology 1998; 208: 521–524.
7. Carty H, Pierce A. Non-accidental injury: a retrospective analysis of a large cohort. Eur Radiol 2002; 12: 2919–2925.
8. Allen WE III, Kier EL, Rothman SL. Pitfalls in the evaluation of skull trauma. A review. Radiol Clin North Am 1973; 11: 479–503.
9. Shapiro R. Anomalous parietal sutures and the bipartite parietal bone. AJR 1972; 115: 569–577.
10. Matsumura G, Uchiumi T, Kida K et al. Developmental studies on the interparietal part of the human occipital squama. J Anat 1993; 182: 197–204.
11. Billmire ME, Myers PA. Serious head injury in infants: accident or abuse? Pediatrics 1985; 75: 340–342.
12. Merten DF, Osborne DRS, Radkowski MA, Leonidas JC. Craniocerebral trauma in the child abuse syndrome: radiologic observations. Pediatr Radiol 1984; 14: 272–277.
13. Lonergan GJ, Baker AM, Morey MK et al. Child abuse: Radiologic–pathologic correlation. Radiographics 2003; 23: 811–845.
14. Worlock P, Stower M, Barbor P. Pattern of fractures in accidental and non-accidental injury in children: a comparative study. Br Med J 1986; 293: 100–102.
15. Gean AD. Non-accidental trauma (child abuse). In: Gean AD, ed. Imaging of head trauma. Raven Press: New York, 1994, 411–426.
16. Hobbs CJ. Skull fracture and the diagnosis of abuse. Arch Dis Child 1984; 59: 246–252.
17. Merten DF, Radkowski MA, Leonidas JC. The abused child: a radiological reappraisal. Radiology 1983; 146: 377–381.
18. Loder RT, Bookout C. Fracture patterns in battered children. J Orthop Trauma 1991; 5: 428–433.
19. King J, Diefendorf D, Apthorp J et al. Analysis of 429 fractures in 189 battered children. J Pediatr Orthop 1988; 8: 585–589.
20. Rao P, Carty H. Non-accidental injury: review of the radiology. Clin Radiol 1999; 54: 11–24.
21. Gilles EE, Nelson MD. Cerebral complications of nonaccidental head injury in childhood. Pediatr Neurol 1998; 19: 119–128.

# 3 FACE

## THE MIDFACE AND ORBIT
The number of routine projections varies between hospitals.

### Common practice
A two-view protocol is common.

- Angled upwards frontal radiograph – the occipitomental (OM) view (Fig. 3.1)
- An OM view with increased upward tilt of the face – the OM 30° view (Fig. 3.2).

### Alternative practice
One OM projection only. Either an OM 30° or an OM15°. A single angled up radiograph will exclude most fractures.[1–3]

### The lateral radiograph ... is redundant.
The superimposition of bones makes the radiographic anatomy on this view difficult to evaluate. In practice, a lateral radiograph rarely adds any important information to the initial assessment of an injury.[4]

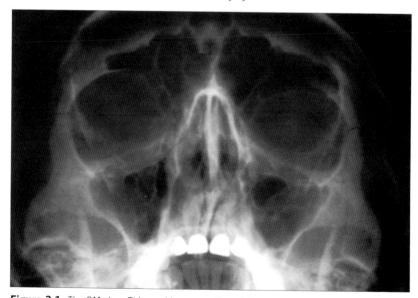

**Figure 3.1** *The OM view. This provides an excellent demonstration of both the upper and middle thirds of the face.*

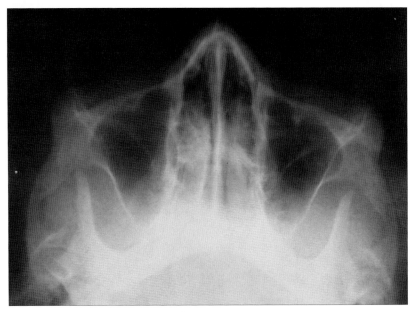

**Figure 3.2** *The OM 30° view. This is the best view for demonstrating the zygomatic arches and the walls of the maxillary antra. The upper third of the face will not be shown well.*

## THE MANDIBLE

■ Most departments have equipment that provides a tomographic 'unwrapped' view of the entire mandible (Fig. 3.3), often referred to as an orthopantomogram (OPG). This panoramic view will show almost all mandibular fractures. Occasionally, fractures through the symphysis menti will not be identified

■ OPG equipment has made routine oblique views of the mandible superfluous. A PA view is occasionally useful for identifying additional sites of fracture when the OPG has already shown one abnormality. The PA view demonstrates the body of the mandible and provides tangential views of the mandibular rami (Fig. 3.4).

## THE NASAL BONE

Referral for radiography is not necessary even if a fracture is certain on clinical examination.[5,6] Radiography is only indicated when requested by a specialist surgeon.

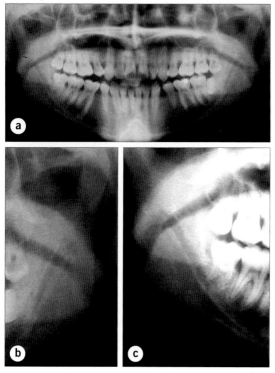

**Figure 3.3** *(a)* *A panoramic (OPG) view of the mandible.* *(b)* *The mandibular condyle is well demonstrated.* *(c)* *Note the common artefact (curved black line) produced by the back of the tongue outlined by air in the pharynx.*

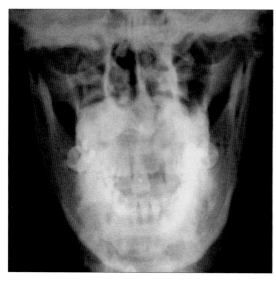

**Figure 3.4** *PA mandible. The condyles are difficult to see because of superimposition of bones. The body of the mandible is displayed well.*

## ANATOMY

On the two occipitomental (OM) projections:

■ The superior and inferior orbital margins, frontal sinuses, zygomatic arches and maxillary antra are visualised with minimal overlap from other bones (Figs 3.1, 3.2)

■ The zygomatic arches, frequent sites of injury, are easy to identify. Each arch may be likened to an elephant's trunk (Fig. 3.5).

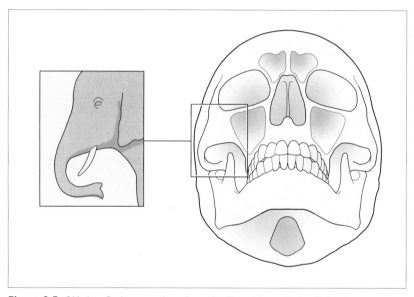

**Figure 3.5** *OM view. Each zygomatic arch can be likened to an elephant's trunk.*

## INJURIES

## A SYSTEM FOR INSPECTING THE OCCIPITOMENTAL VIEW

Fractures of the middle third of the face are commonly classified according to the Le Fort fracture patterns. This is useful to maxillofacial surgeons when planning treatment.

In practice, the Le Fort classification is not particularly helpful when carrying out a step-by-step assessment of the radiographs in the Emergency Department. A simpler approach – the McGrigor concept – is recommended.

McGrigor described how an OM view can be assessed by utilising a series of lines traced over the radiograph.[7] The following is a modified version of the McGrigor concept.

### McGrigor's three lines

■ Trace each line on the OM view (Figs 3.6, 3.7)

■ As each line is traced, the injured side is compared with the uninjured side

■ The soft tissues above and below each line should be scrutinised. A fluid level, or a maxillary antrum containing a soft tissue opacity, may indicate that there is an underlying fracture.

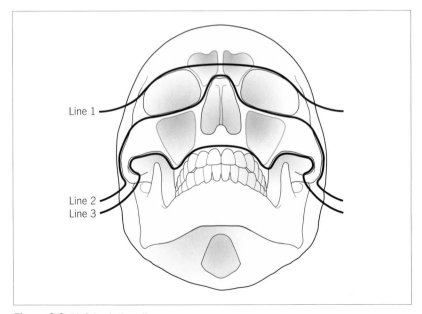

**Figure 3.6** *McGrigor's three lines.*

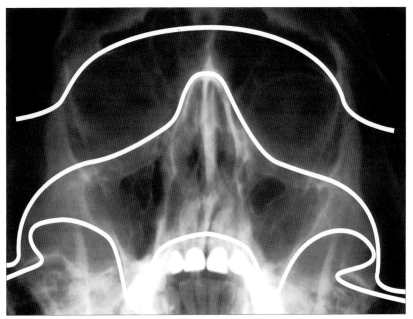

**Figure 3.7** *Normal OM, showing McGrigor's lines. Line 1 (top), Line 2 (middle), Line 3 (bottom).*

## LINE 1

Starting outside the face:

- Trace the line through the synchondrosis (i.e. the suture) between the frontal bone and the zygomatic bone at the lateral margin of the orbit (RED LINE)

- Follow across the forehead, assessing the superior orbital margin and the frontal sinus (BLUE LINE)

- Continue on to the other side of the radiograph following the same landmarks (Figs 3.8, 3.9) (GREEN LINE)

- The injured and uninjured sides should be compared

- Always correlate the radiological findings with the clinical signs.

### *Look for:*

- Fractures

- Widening of the zygomatico-frontal suture

- Fluid level (haemorrhage) in a frontal sinus.

---

**Pitfall:** The width of the normal zygomatico-frontal suture varies between individuals. Compare the injured with the uninjured side.

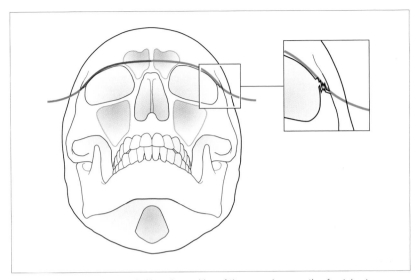

**Figure 3.8** *McGrigor's line 1. Note the position of the normal zygomatico-frontal suture.*

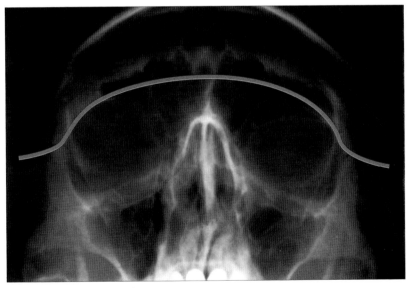

**Figure 3.9** *McGrigor's line 1.*

## LINE 2

Starting outside the face:

■ Trace a line upwards along the superior border of the zygomatic arch (up the elephant's trunk) crossing the body of the zygoma (RED LINE)

■ Continue on to the inferior margin of the orbit and over the bridge of the nose (BLUE LINE)

■ Follow the same landmarks on to the other side of the face (Figs 3.10, 3.11) (GREEN LINE).

### *Look for:*

■ Fractures of the zygomatic arch (Fig. 3.12)

■ A fracture through the inferior rim of the orbit

■ A soft tissue shadow in the roof of the maxillary antrum (see page 60 blow-out fracture).

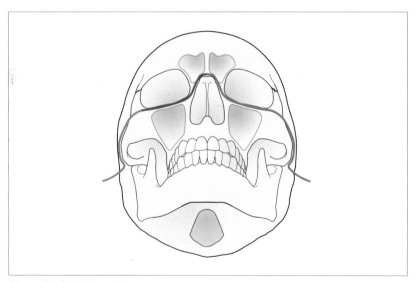

**Figure 3.10** *McGrigor's line 2.*

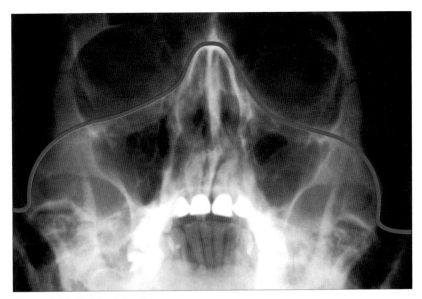

**Figure 3.11** *McGrigor's line 2.*

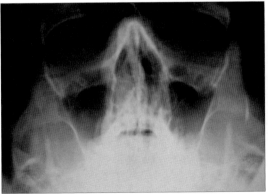

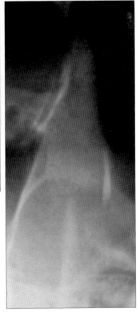

**Figure 3.12** *Tracing McGrigor's line 2 reveals a step (fracture) in the normal curve of the left zygomatic arch (elephant's trunk). Compare this with the appearance of the uninjured right zygomatic arch.*

## LINE 3

Starting outside the face:

- Trace a line along the inferior margin of the zygomatic arch (under the elephant's trunk) (RED LINE)

- Down the lateral wall of the maxillary antrum (BLUE LINE)

- Continue along the inferior margin of the antrum, across the maxilla, including the roots of the upper teeth (look very carefully – fractures of this part of the maxilla are extremely difficult to detect) (BLUE LINE)

- Follow the same structures on to the other side of the face (Figs 3.13, 3.14) (GREEN LINE).

***Look for:***

- Fractures of the zygoma and of the lateral aspect of the maxillary antrum (Fig. 3.15)

- A fluid level in the maxillary antrum. In the context of trauma – assume that a fluid level represents haemorrhage from a fracture (Fig. 3.16).

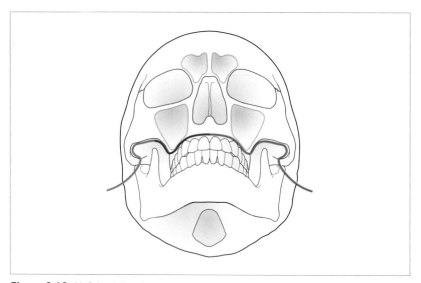

**Figure 3.13** *McGrigor's line 3.*

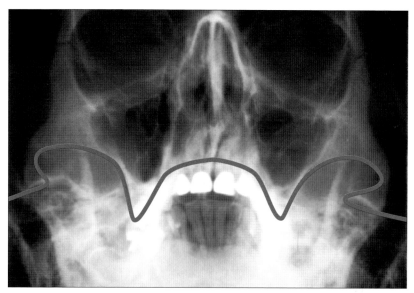

**Figure 3.14** *McGrigor's line 3.*

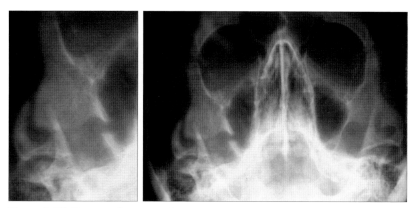

**Figure 3.15** *Tracing McGrigor's line 3 reveals fractures of the right zygomatic arch and of the lateral wall of the maxillary antrum.*

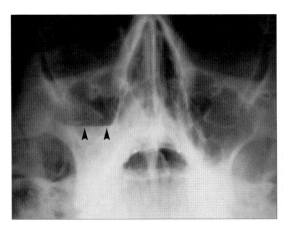

**Figure 3.16** *Fluid level in the right maxillary antrum. Following trauma this is most likely to be blood from a fracture. The fracture is not visible on this radiograph.*

## PARTICULAR INJURIES

### The midface

■ An isolated fracture of the zygomatic arch is common

■ Isolated fractures through the zygomatico-frontal suture, or through the body of the zygoma, are rare

■ Fractures often occur as part of a combination injury known as a *tripod fracture* (Fig. 3.17). This comprises:

**1** Widening of the zygomatico-frontal suture

**2** A fracture of the zygomatic arch

**3** A fracture through the body of the zygoma. This particular fracture is seen as a break in the inferior margin of the orbit and a break in the lateral wall of the maxillary antrum (Figs 3.17 and 3.18).

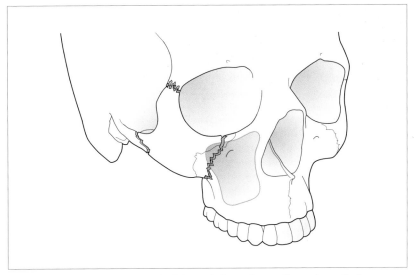

**Figure 3.17** *Tripod fracture. The shaded area indicates the maxillary antrum. On the OM radiograph the fracture through the body of the zygoma will appear as fractures through the inferior wall of the orbit and through the lateral wall of the maxillary antrum.*

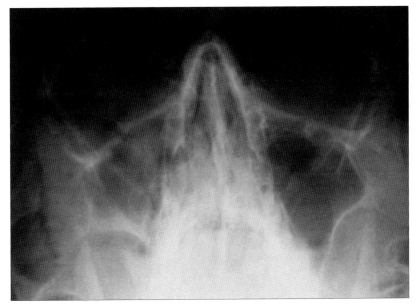

**Figure 3.18** *Right tripod fracture.*

## The orbital margin

- This is made up of strong, thick bones that protect the orbital contents
- Fractures of the orbital margin may occur in isolation or may be part of a more complicated fracture such as a tripod fracture
- An isolated fracture of the margin usually involves the inferior and lateral aspect.

## The orbital walls: blow-out fractures

- May be:
  - Isolated
  - Part of a combination injury[8,9]
- Result from a direct compressive force to the globe, commonly from a fist or a small object such as a squash ball (Fig. 3.19)
- A bone abnormality is rarely seen unless a blow-out fracture is accompanied by an additional injury to the mid face. These combination injuries do occur. Nevertheless, an isolated or pure blow-out fracture is common
- With an isolated blow-out fracture:
  - The strong inferior orbital rim (i.e. margin) remains intact
  - The walls fracture at the weakest points. These are the thin plates of bone that form the floor of the orbit (i.e. the roof of the maxillary antrum) and the medial wall of the orbit (i.e. the lateral margin of the ethmoid sinus)
  - Some of the orbital contents may herniate downwards through the orbital floor (Figs 3.19–3.21). This has been likened to an opaque teardrop hanging from the roof of the antrum. The teardrop may be the only radiographic evidence of a blow-out fracture. It should be detected when McGrigor's second line is traced
  - The depressed bone fragment from the orbital floor is often rotated. As a consequence it is usually very difficult to identify
  - Sometimes the fracture through the wall of the maxillary or ethmoid sinus may only be inferred because air from a sinus has entered the orbit. The air may be seen on the radiograph above the globe, giving rise to the term 'the black eyebrow sign' (Fig. 3.22)
  - The pattern of abnormalities will vary between individual patients. One, some or all of these signs may be present (Fig. 3.23).

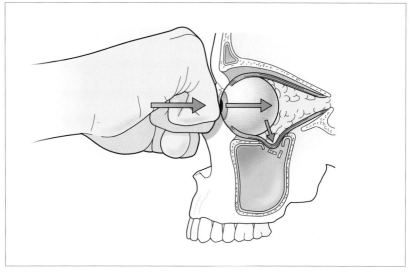

**Figure 3.19** *Blow-out fracture. Increased intraorbital pressure has caused a fracture of the thin plate of bone that forms the floor of the orbit. Fat and muscle have herniated downwards, resulting in an appearance rather like a teardrop in the roof of the maxillary antrum.*

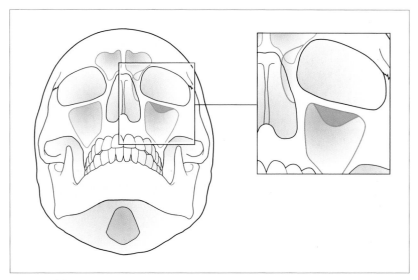

**Figure 3.20** *Blow-out fracture. The soft tissue teardrop in the roof of the maxillary antrum represents herniated orbital contents (dark shading). Herniation through the medial wall of the orbit into the ethmoid sinus (light shading) commonly occurs but is difficult to detect on the radiographs.*

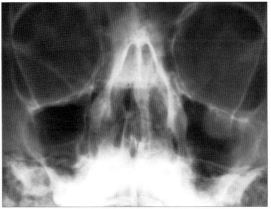

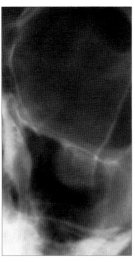

**Figure 3.21** *Blow out fracture. Soft tissue (the teardrop) is seen hanging from the roof of the left maxillary antrum.*

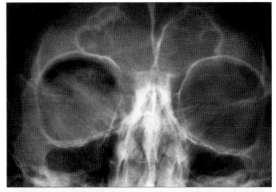

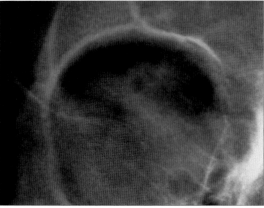

**Figure 3.22** *Blow-out fracture. The radiographic appearances are entirely within normal limits, apart from the black eyebrow sign. This appearance is due to air from a sinus entering the orbit.*

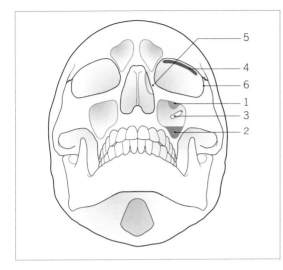

**Figure 3.23** *Isolated blow-out fractures. All, some or none of the following may be seen: 1 = tear drop in antrum, 2 = fluid level in antrum, 3 = thin plate of bone from the orbital floor displaced into the antrum, 4 = black eyebrow sign, 5 = opaque (blood filled) ethmoid sinus.*

## The mandible

■ The mandible should be regarded as a rigid ring of bone. When a bone ring is broken it is very common for two fractures to occur (Figs 3.24, 3.25)

■ Approximately 50% of mandibular fractures are bilateral

■ Fractures of the body and angle of the mandible are particularly common (Figs 3.24, 3.25)

■ The mandibular condyles must be carefully scrutinised. Fractures occur frequently at these sites. They may be very subtle

■ It is particularly important that the radiological evaluation is correlated with the precise site of clinical injury.

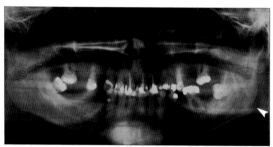

**Figure 3.24**
Orthopantomogram. This panoramic view shows a fracture through the body of the mandible on the right side. There is a second fracture through the left angle of the mandible.

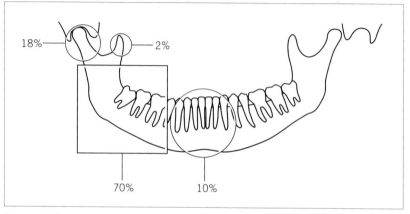

**Figure 3.25** Fractures of the mandible. Site incidence. Note the dislocation of the left temporo-mandibular joint.

**Pitfall 1:** Occasionally, the panoramic view (OPG) will fail to show a fracture.[8] The symphysis is a particularly difficult site. A near-normal appearance can occur when the fragments override each other. Clinical correlation/suspicion must apply even when the OPG view appears normal. When the OPG appears normal but strong clinical suspicion of a fracture remains, a PA view can be very helpful in providing reassurance/further information (Fig. 3.26).

**Pitfall 2:** To the inexperienced, the panoramic view will produce appearances that can be confused with a fracture. These artefacts are due to the overlapping image of the pharynx or tongue (Fig. 3.3). Familiarity with the normal appearances will prevent incorrect interpretation.

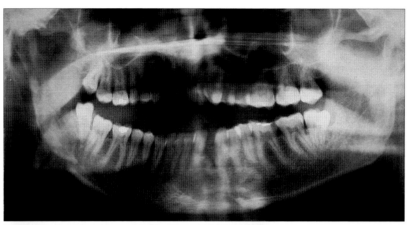

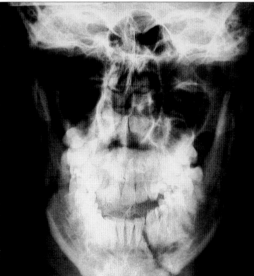

**Figure 3.26** *The orthopantomogram clearly shows two fractures. The PA view reveals a third fracture through the left condyle. Remember – the OPG does not always show all fractures. Clinical suspicion will dictate whether an additional radiograph (such as a PA view) should be obtained in order to clear a site that remains clinically worrying.*

## KEY POINTS

### INJURIES TO THE MIDFACE AND ORBIT
#### Concentrate on the OM views

- Note the *elephant's trunk* appearance of each zygomatic arch

- Trace the three McGrigor's lines. Look for bone and soft tissue abnormalities

- Compare the injured side with the normal side

- Tripod fracture: if you see any one of the components of this fracture complex then look for the other associated fractures

- With an isolated blow-out fracture look for a soft-tissue teardrop in the roof of the maxillary antrum. Do not expect to see a bone abnormality.

### INJURIES TO THE MANDIBLE

- Regard the mandible as a bone ring. Solitary fractures do occur – but two fractures are common

- The panoramic (OPG) view detects almost all fractures – but the sensitivity is not 100%. If clinical worry persists, the radiologist will arrange for additional views to be obtained.

### INJURIES TO THE NOSE

- Radiography is not indicated in the Emergency Department.

## THE SUBTLE SIGN NOT TO MISS

| Radiograph | Appearance | Significance |
| --- | --- | --- |
| OM view | The 'black eyebrow' sign | A blow-out fracture of the orbit, i.e. the roof of the maxillary antrum or the medial wall of the ethmoid sinus has been fractured and air has entered the orbit. |

# REFERENCES

1. Sidebottom AJ, Sissons G. Radiographic screening for midfacial fracture in A and E. Br J Radiol 1999; 72: 523–524.
2. McGhee A, Guse J. Radiography for midfacial trauma: is a single OM15° radiograph as sensitive as OM15° and OM30° combined? Br J Radiol 2000; 73: 883–885.
3. Pogrel MA, Podlesh SW, Goldman KE. Efficacy of a single occipitomental radiograph to screen for midfacial fractures. J Oral Maxillofacial Surg 2000; 58: 24–26.
4. Raby N, Moore D. Radiography of facial trauma: the lateral view is not required. Clin Radiol 1998; 53: 218–220.
5. de Lacey GJ, Wignall BK, Hussain S, Reidy JR. The radiology of nasal injuries: problems of interpretation and clinical relevance. Br J Radiol 1977; 50: 412–414.
6. Li S, Papsin B, Braun DH. Value of nasal radiographs in nasal trauma management. J Otolaryngol 1996; 25: 162–164.
7. McGrigor DB, Campbell W. The radiology of war injuries. Part VI. Wounds of the face and jaw. Br J Radiol 1950; 23: 685–696.
8. Druelinger L, Guenther M, Marchand EG. Radiographic evaluation of the facial complex. Emerg Med Clin North Am 2000; 18: 393–410.
9. Hammerschlag SB, Hughes S, O'Reilly GV et al. Blow-out fractures of the orbit: a comparison of computed tomography and conventional radiography with anatomical correlation. Radiology 1982; 143: 487–492.

# 4 SHOULDER

## BASIC RADIOGRAPHS

- An AP projection (Fig. 4.1) is standard in all hospitals
- The second projection will vary. There are three options.

**Table 4.1** Options for the second projection

| Option | Advantages | Disadvantages |
|---|---|---|
| Axial (= armpit view; Figs 4.2, 4.3) | ■ Common practice <br> ■ Technique well understood by radiographers <br> ■ Will show fragments detached from the glenoid or from the head of the humerus | ■ Abduction of the injured arm is essential and can be very painful <br> ■ Pain may prevent a technically good radiograph from being obtained <br> ■ Poor technique = difficult to interpret |
| Lateral scapular radiograph (= Y view; Figs 4.2, 4.4) | ■ Technically easy <br> ■ No discomfort to the patient <br> ■ Easy to interpret | ■ Small detached fragments (from the glenoid or the head of humerus) often not shown |
| Apical oblique (= modified armpit view; Figs 4.2, 4.5) | ■ Patient's arm not moved <br> ■ No discomfort to the patient <br> ■ Very easy to interpret <br> ■ Small bone fragments well shown | ■ Underused <br> ■ Some radiographers and radiologists are unfamiliar with the projection – this is the only disadvantage |

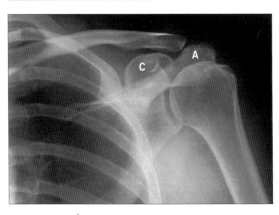

**Figure 4.1** *The AP view. A = acromion, C = coracoid.*

Axial

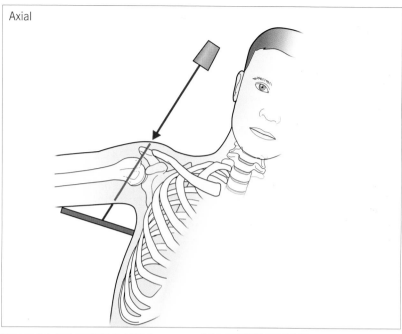

Y

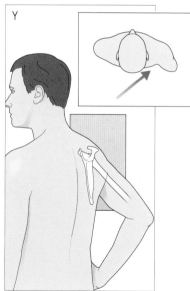

Apical oblique

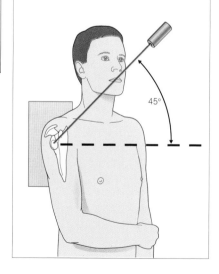

45°

**Figure 4.2**  *Radiographic technique.*

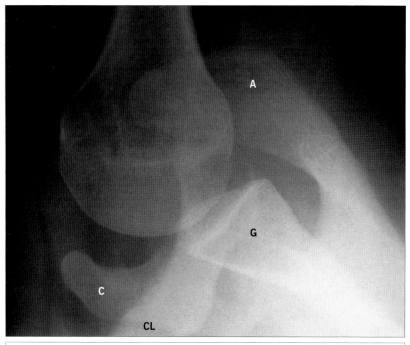

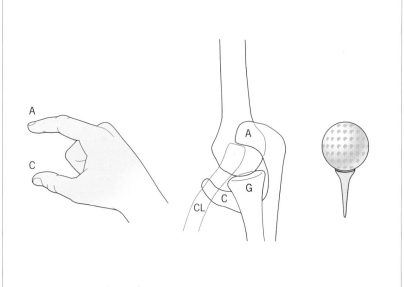

**Figure 4.3** *The axial or armpit view. A = acromion; C = coracoid; G = glenoid; CL = clavicle. The head of the humerus sits on the glenoid like a golf ball on a tee. Orientation is easy: the 'fingers' (i.e. the acromion (A) and coracoid (C) processes) always point anteriorly.*

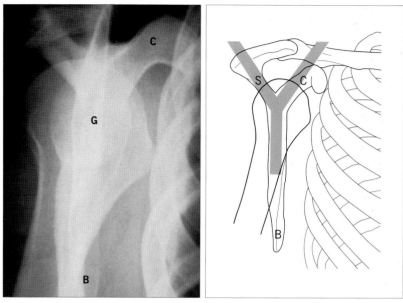

**Figure 4.4** *Lateral scapular or the Y view. The humeral head overlies the centre of the glenoid (G). The Y is formed by the junction of the edge of the scapular blade (B), the coracoid (C) and the spine of the scapula (S).*

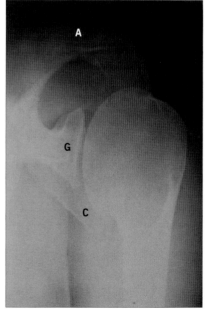

**Figure 4.5** *The apical oblique view or the modified armpit view. A = acromion; C = coracoid; G = glenoid.*

## ANTEROPOSTERIOR PROJECTION

■ The humeral head is not round and symmetrical. It has a configuration that mimics the head of a walking stick (Figs 4.1, 4.6)

**Note:** the walking stick appearance is due to positioning the humerus in external rotation when the AP radiograph is obtained. This positioning has a relevance to the diagnosis of true and false posterior dislocations (see Pitfall, p. 84).

■ The articular surfaces of the humerus and the glenoid parallel each other (Figs 4.1, 4.6)

■ The inferior cortices of the acromion process and the clavicle should align (Figs 4.1, 4.7). A proper assessment usually requires the use of a bright light or appropriate windowing.

## AXIAL (ARMPIT) PROJECTION

In order to make interpretation easier the radiograph should be orientated so that the glenoid resembles a golf tee.

■ The humerus sits on the glenoid like a golf ball on the tee (Fig. 4.3)

■ The acromion and coracoid processes can be likened to fingers pointing forwards/anteriorly.

## Y PROJECTION[1-3]

Evaluate the radiograph (Fig. 4.4) by looking directly into the glenoid.

■ Anterior is on the side of the rib cage

■ The stem of the Y is the blade of the scapula

■ The limbs of the Y are the coracoid and the spine of the scapula, the latter merging with the acromion process

■ The junction formed by the stem and the limbs of the Y indicate the centre of the glenoid

■ The centre of the head of the humerus should overlap the junction formed by the stem and limbs of the Y.

## APICAL OBLIQUE PROJECTION[4,5]

This shows the glenohumeral joint and the bones very clearly (Fig. 4.5).

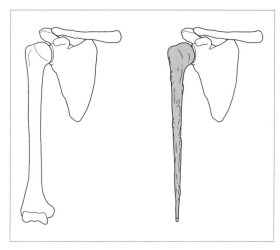

**Figure 4.6** On the AP projection the normal humeral head has a configuration rather like that of a club-headed walking stick.

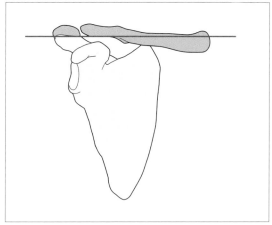

**Figure 4.7** Normal acromioclavicular joint. The most common alignment is shown.

## NORMAL VARIANTS

■ On the AP projection, in the immature skeleton, the growth plate for the head of the humerus lies obliquely. It appears as two lucent lines (Fig. 4.8). Either of these lines may be mistaken for a fracture

■ The tips of the acromion and the coracoid processes ossify from separate centres. In children these appear as separate pieces of bone and may also be mistaken for fracture fragments – especially on the axial or armpit view (Fig. 4.9). Occasionally these centres persist into adulthood.

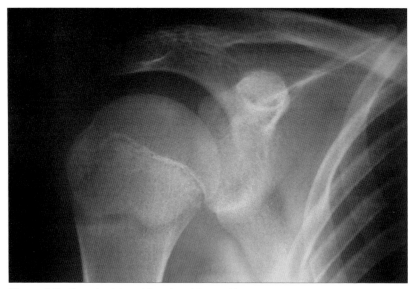

**Figure 4.8** *Normal epiphyseal lines in a 14-year-old.*

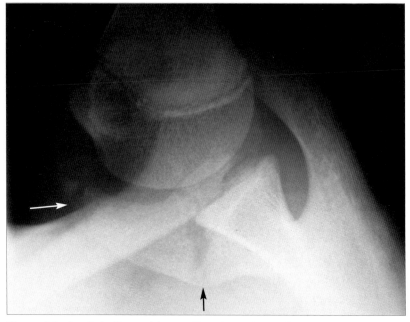

**Figure 4.9** *Armpit view in an adolescent. Normal secondary ossification centre (white arrow) at the tip of the coracoid and an epiphyseal line at the base of the coracoid (black arrow). These appearances may be mistaken for fractures.*

INJURIES

## FRACTURES AND DISLOCATIONS – COMMON

- Through the neck of the humerus and its greater tuberosity (Fig. 4.10)

- Involving the head of the humerus and/or the glenoid rim. These are common complications of an anterior dislocation (Figs 4.11, 4.12)

- Clavicle. The position of the fracture is usually age related. Under 20 years the majority of fractures involve the middle third. Lateral third fractures[6] dominate after the age of 20 (Fig. 4.13).

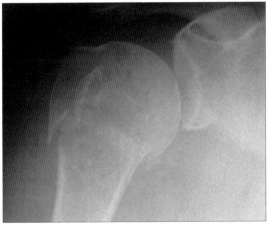

**Figure 4.10** *A comminuted fracture involving the surgical neck and the greater tuberosity of the humerus.*

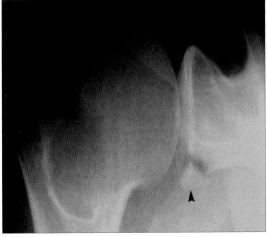

**Figure 4.11** *A common complication of an anterior dislocation: fracture of the glenoid shown on this apical oblique projection (arrowed).*

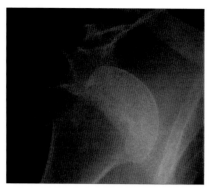

**Figure 4.12** *A common complication of an anterior dislocation: fracture of the greater tuberosity of the humerus.*

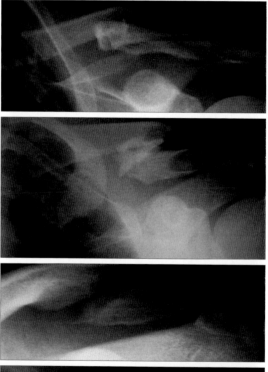

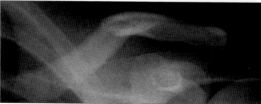

**Figure 4.13** *Clavicle fractures. Most fractures involve the middle third; a few involve the outer third; most are easy to detect; some are slightly more difficult to detect.*

## ANTERIOR DISLOCATION

- Very common. Over 95% of glenohumeral dislocations

- The following appearances are characteristic (Figs 4.14–4.17):

  - ❏ The head of the humerus lies under the coracoid process on the AP view

  - ❏ The armpit and the apical oblique views show the golf ball (head of the humerus) anterior to the tee (glenoid)

  - ❏ The Y view shows the head of the humerus to be displaced anteriorly. It no longer covers the glenoid (the centre of the Y).

**Note:**

- Both projections should always be examined for a fragment detached from the glenoid rim or from the posterior aspect of the head of the humerus (Figs 4.11, 4.12). These associated fractures are common. If a fragment enters the joint it may prevent a successful reduction

- The associated common fractures or deformities are often described eponymously

  - ❏ The Hill–Sachs deformity is a compression fracture of the posterolateral aspect of the humeral head

  - ❏ Bankart's lesion is a fracture of the anterior lip of the glenoid

- Following manipulation, a repeat AP view should always be obtained in order to confirm that reduction has occurred.

---

**Pitfall:** Pseudosubluxation. Following an injury, haemorrhage into the joint may push the head of the humerus inferiorly. The head of the humerus does not move medially. The inferior displacement can be misinterpreted as a dislocation (Fig. 4.18). The haemorrhage distending the joint will absorb and the pseudosubluxation will disappear within a week or two.

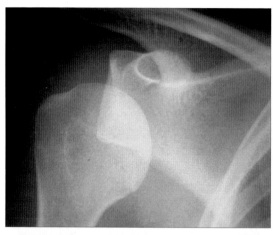

**Figure 4.14** *Anterior dislocation. Typical appearance on the AP radiograph. The subcoracoid position of the humeral head is characteristic.*

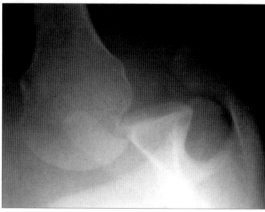

**Figure 4.15** *Anterior dislocation. Axial (armpit) view. The humeral head (the golf ball) lies anterior to the glenoid (the tee). The acromion process and the coracoid (the fingers) point anteriorly.*

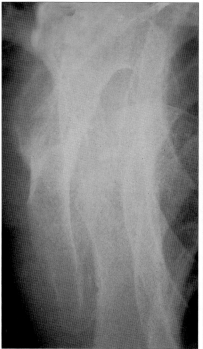

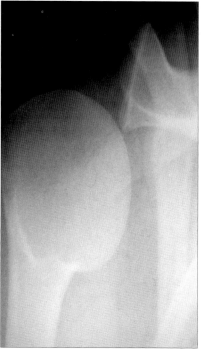

**Figure 4.16** *Anterior dislocation. Y view. The humeral head lies anterior to the glenoid – the centre of the Y.*

**Figure 4.17** *Anterior dislocation. Oblique axial view. The humeral head lies anterior to the glenoid. (Compare this appearance with the normal position of the humeral head in Figure 4.5.)*

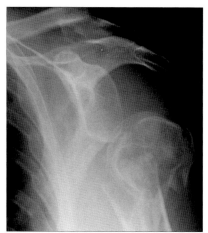

**Figure 4.18** *Pitfall: Not a dislocation. Comminuted fracture of the surgical neck of the humerus. The head of the humerus is displaced inferiorly but not anteriorly. This displacement is caused by haemorrhage into the joint, which pushes the head of the humerus downwards. The second view will confirm that the head of the humerus is not positioned anteriorly nor posteriorly. The humeral head will return to an anatomical position within a few days as the large haemarthrosis resolves.*

## FRACTURES AND DISLOCATIONS – UNCOMMON

### Scapula

These fractures are easy to over look (Fig. 4.19). Both radiographic projections must be scrutinised very carefully.

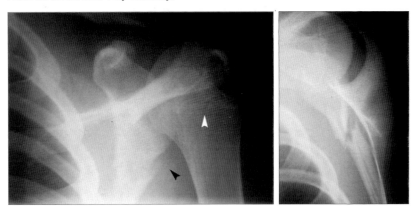

**Figure 4.19** *Adolescent. Normal gleno-humeral joint. The fracture through the body of the scapula was overlooked (black arrow). Normal epiphyseal line (white arrow).*

## POSTERIOR DISLOCATION

- Uncommon. Fewer than 5% of shoulder dislocations. 50% are overlooked on the initial radiographs[7,8]

- Often results from severe muscle spasm, either during a convulsion or electric shock

- The following appearances are characteristic (Figs 4.20–4.23):

  - ❏ *On the AP view* the humeral head frequently appears symmetrical or rounded in appearance. This has been likened to a light bulb. The light bulb appearance is due to the humerus being internally rotated. An inability to externally rotate the upper arm is a characteristic feature of this injury

  - ❏ *On the Y view* the centre of the head of the humerus lies posterior to the junction of the limbs of the Y

  - ❏ *On the axial (armpit) and on the apical oblique view* the golf ball (head of the humerus) lies posterior to the tee (glenoid).

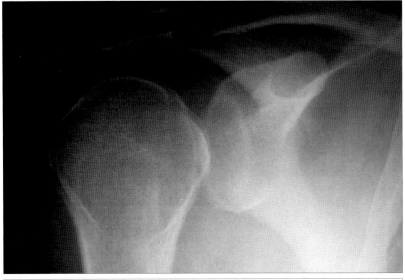

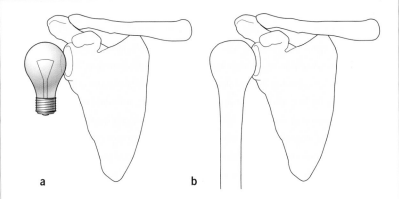

**Figure 4.20** *Posterior dislocation.* **(a)** *AP view. The head of the humerus often (but not always) adopts the shape of a light bulb* **(b)**. *It no longer resembles the head of a club-headed walking stick.*

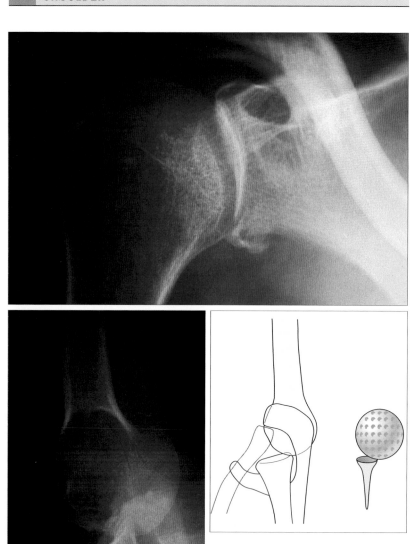

**Figure 4.21** *Posterior dislocation. In this patient the humeral head resembles a walking stick on the AP view. However, on the axial (armpit) view the humeral head lies posterior to the glenoid – the golf ball is off the tee.*

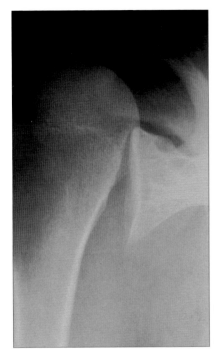

**Figure 4.22** *Posterior dislocation. Oblique axial view. The head of the humerus lies posterior to the glenoid.*

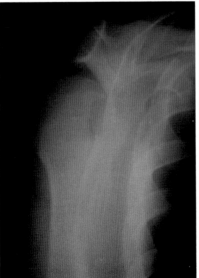 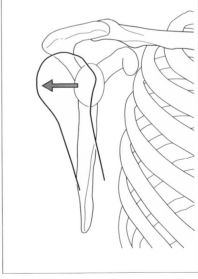

**Figure 4.23** *Posterior dislocation. Y view. The humeral head lies behind the glenoid (the centre of the Y).*

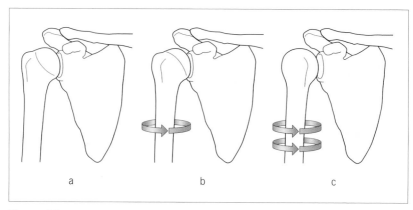

a          b          c

**Figure 4.24** *Pitfall: the effect of internal rotation on the contour of the humeral head. Standard AP radiographs are always obtained with the humerus positioned in slight external rotation and this accounts for the humeral head looking like a club-headed walking stick as shown in (a). However, the injured joint may be so painful that the patient holds the arm in internal rotation. When this occurs then a light bulb appearance (b, c) may result and can mimic a posterior dislocation. An error in interpretation will be avoided by checking the precise position of the head of the humerus on the second view.*

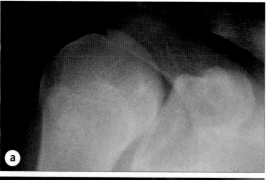

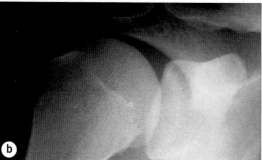

**Figure 4.25** *Pitfall: the light bulb appearance of the head of the humerus (a) is not due to a posterior dislocation. It is due to pain causing the upper arm to be held in a position of internal rotation. A repeat film (b) was obtained with the shoulder correctly radiographed with some degree of external rotation – the normal walking stick appearance is now present.*

## ACROMIOCLAVICULAR JOINT INJURY

■ A very common injury

■ Evaluate this joint on the AP view of the shoulder

■ Do not evaluate the acromioclavicular (A-C) joint on any of the other projections, as the appearance can be confusing

■ The width of the normal joint is very variable and depends in part on the angle of radiographic projection. In the context of trauma a width of 8 mm or more should be viewed with suspicion – but 8–10 mm can be normal in some adults

■ The key observation: the inferior cortex of the acromion process and the inferior cortex of the clavicle should align (Figs 4.26, 4.27)

■ Subluxation is detected as a step between the inferior cortices of the acromion process and the clavicle (Figs 4.26, 4.28)

■ Sometimes the radiographic appearance will be equivocal. In these patients joint separation will be revealed (or excluded) if an AP radiograph of both shoulders is obtained while the patient holds a weight in each hand. This allows comparison between the injured and the uninjured side (Fig. 4.27).

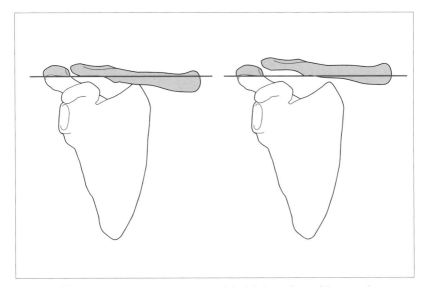

**Figure 4.26** *Normal and abnormal alignment of the inferior surfaces of the acromion process and the clavicle. Normal on the left, subluxation on the right.*

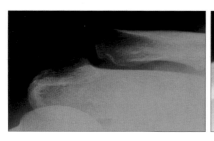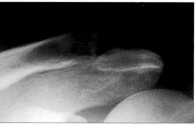

**Figure 4.27** *AP radiograph of both shoulders obtained with a weight held in each hand. Normal alignment of the left acromioclavicular joint; subluxation at the right acromioclavicular joint.*

## CORACOCLAVICULAR LIGAMENT INJURY

The normal distance between the coracoid and the clavicle on the AP view is less than 1.3 cm.[9,10]

- If rupture of these ligaments is a clinical concern, weight-bearing views of both sides are indicated (Table 4.2)

- A difference of 5 mm or more in the distance between the coracoid and the clavicle on the injured compared with the normal side indicates a rupture of the ligaments.

**Table 4.2** Injury to the ligaments anchoring the scapula to the clavicle[11]

| Grade of injury | Damage | Radiological findings | Usual treatment |
|---|---|---|---|
| I | ■ Stretching or partial rupture of the A-C ligament but intact coracoclavicular ligaments | ■ Normal or slight step at the AC joint | ■ Conservative |
| II | ■ Rupture of the A-C ligament and stretching of the coracoclavicular ligaments | ■ A step at the AC joint – may need stress views if equivocal | ■ Conservative Occasionally surgical |
| III | ■ Rupture of the acromioclavicular ligaments and rupture of the coracoclavicular ligament | ■ A step at the AC joint Increased coracoclavicular distance (i.e. greater than 1.3 cm). May need stress views to show the full extent of the damage | ■ Surgical |

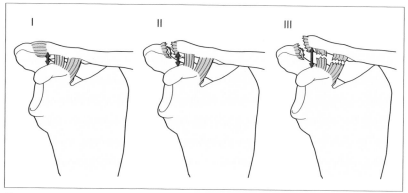

**Figure 4.28** *Acromioclavicular joint injuries are classified on the basis of the extent of the injury to the acromioclavicular (AC) and coracoclavicular (CC) ligaments (see Table 4.2). Type I: AC ligaments stretched but intact. CC ligaments normal. The coracoclavicular distance (arrow) is normal. This distance should be less than 1.3 cm. Type II: AC ligaments completely torn. CC ligaments stretched but intact. The coracoclavicular distance (arrow) remains within normal limits. Type III: Both the AC and the CC ligaments are completely torn. The coracoclavicular distance (arrow) is abnormal.*

## KEY POINTS

- Scrutinise both views: 'assessing one view only is one view too few'

- Understand the normal anatomy on the local second view

- Anterior dislocation. Diagnosis is easy. Look for fracture fragments. Always request a postreduction film to check that reduction has been achieved

- Posterior dislocation. As many as 50% are missed in the Emergency Department. Suspect this diagnosis if the humeral head appears rounded or like a light bulb. Diagnosis is easy when the normal anatomy on the second view is properly understood

- A-C joint. The inferior cortices of the acromion process and the clavicle should align on the AP radiograph.

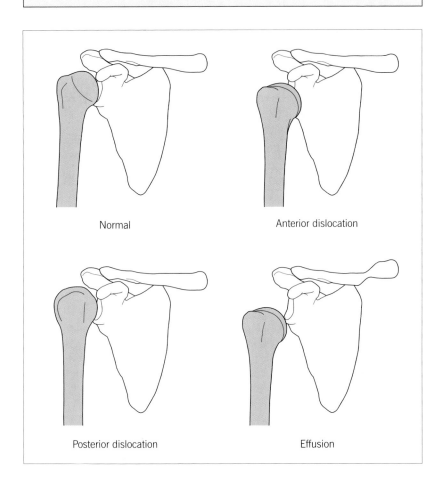

Normal

Anterior dislocation

Posterior dislocation

Effusion

## THE SUBTLE SIGN NOT TO MISS

| Radiograph | Sign | Significance |
| --- | --- | --- |
| AP | The space between the coracoid process and the clavicle exceeds 1.3 cm | ■ Rupture of the coracoclavicular ligaments<br>■ Surgery often required |

## REFERENCES

1. Rubin SA, Gray RL, Green WR. The shoulder 'Y': a diagnostic aid in shoulder trauma. Radiology 1974; 110: 725–726.
2. Horsfield D, Jones SN. A useful projection in radiography of the shoulder. J Bone Joint Surg 1987; 69B: 338.
3. De Smet AA. Anterior oblique projection in radiography of the traumatized shoulder. AJR 1980; 134: 515–518.
4. Kornguth PJ, Salazar AM. The apical oblique view of the shoulder: its usefulness in acute trauma. AJR 1987, 149: 113–116.
5. Garth WP Jr, Slappey CE, Ochs CW. Roentgenographic demonstration of instability of the shoulder: the apical oblique projection. J Bone Joint Surg 1984; 66A: 1450–1453.
6. Stanley D, Norris SH. Recovery following fractures of the clavicle treated conservatively. Injury 1988; 19: 162–164.
7. Hawkins RJ, Neer CS, Pianta RM et al. Locked posterior dislocation of the shoulder. J Bone Joint Surg 1987; 69A: 9–18.
8. Rowe CR, Zarins B. Chronic unreduced dislocations of the shoulder. J Bone and Joint Surg 1982; 64-A: 494–505.
9. Rogers LF. Radiology of skeletal trauma. New York: Churchill Livingstone, 1982.
10. Newstadter LM, Weiss MJ. Trauma to the shoulder girdle. Semin Roentgenol 1991; 26: 331–343.
11. Mlasowsky B, Brenner P, Duben W, Heymann H. Repair of complete acromioclavicular dislocation (Tossy Stage III) using Balser's hook plate combined with ligament sutures. Injury 1988; 19: 162–164.

# 5 ELBOW

## BASIC RADIOGRAPHS

- AP in full extension
- Lateral with 90° of flexion
- Optional – but routine in some departments – the radial head–capitellum view.[1] This view projects the proximal radius away from the other bones. It is an excellent view for evaluating the radial head. **Technique:** the patient is positioned as for the lateral view but the tube is angled 45° to the joint.

## ANATOMY

### ANTEROPOSTERIOR PROJECTION

- The olecranon is obscured by the humerus (Fig. 5.1)
- The capitellum is lateral and articulates with the radial head
- The trochlea is medial and articulates with the ulna
- Note: the external epicondyle in children can be normal but seemingly widely separate from the humerus. However, when normal, its lateral border is always parallel to the cortex of the adjacent humeral metaphysis.

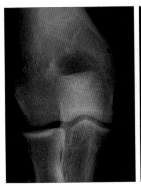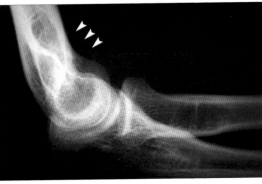

**Figure 5.1** *Normal AP and lateral radiographs. The normally positioned anterior fat pad (arrows) is slightly darker than the surrounding muscle.*

## LATERAL PROJECTION – THE BONES

- The capitellum and trochlea are superimposed
- The radiocapitellar line (Figs 5.2, 5.3) passes through the capitellum
- The anterior humeral line (Fig. 5.4) should have at least one third of the capitellum anterior to it.

## LATERAL PROJECTION – THE SOFT TISSUES

- **Elbow fat pads.** There are two pads of fat related to the distal humerus – anterior and posterior. They are extrasynovial but intracapsular. The fat is in contact with the joint capsule
  - ❏ Fat is seen as a darker streak in the surrounding grey soft tissues
  - ❏ The anterior fat pad will be seen in most (but not all) normal elbows and is characteristically closely applied to the humerus (Figs 5.1, 5.5)
  - ❏ The posterior fat pad is not visible in the normal elbow
- **Supinator fat stripe.** A linear strip of fat overlies the supinator muscle and is positioned anterior to the radial head and neck. It is often claimed that, if this stripe is displaced or obliterated, then there is haemorrhage in the deep soft tissues. A definite association with an occult fracture remains unproven.

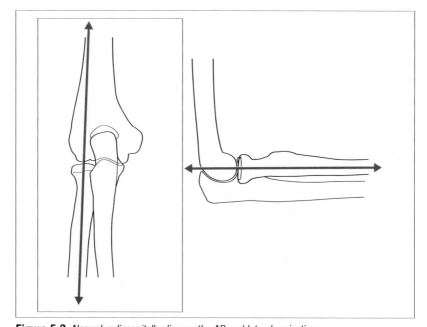

**Figure 5.2** *Normal radiocapitellar line on the AP and lateral projections.*

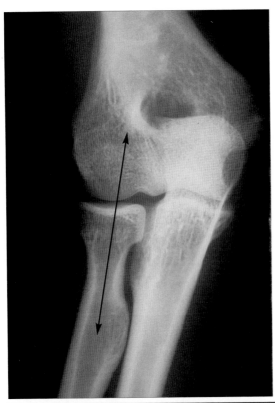

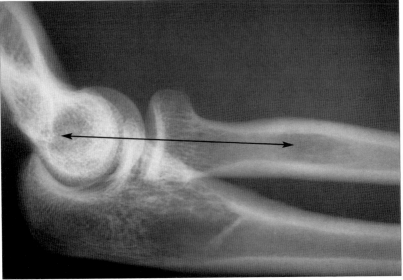

**Figure 5.3** *The normal radiocapitellar line. Note: on the AP view the line is drawn along the centre of the proximal portion of the radius.*

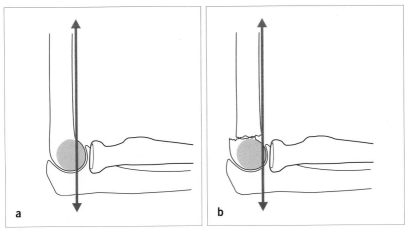

**Figure 5.4** *The anterior humeral line.* **(a)** *In most normal patients approximately one third of the capitellum (shaded) lies anterior to this line.* **(b)** *A supracondylar fracture often results in the distal fragment being displaced posteriorly; as a consequence less than one third of the capitellum may lie anterior to the line.*

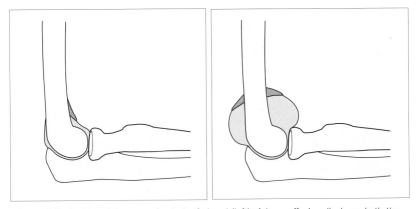

**Figure 5.5** *Position of the normal anterior fad pad (left). A large effusion displaces both the anterior and posterior fat pads away from the humerus (right).*

## INJURIES

- Fractures, dislocations and apophyseal avulsions can be subtle and will be overlooked unless a step-by-step approach is taken when assessing the radiographs

- Pulled (or nursemaid's) elbow in a child. The history is typical – the extended forearm is pulled suddenly

  - ❏ The injury is usually described as being caused by stretching of the annular ligament, which slips proximally on the radial head. Ultrasound[2] demonstrates that the injury is actually due to subluxation of the radial head on to the superior rim of a shallow depression in the adjacent ulna (Fig. 5.6). The conventional explanation that the proximal radius subluxes distally through a stretched annular ligament is mistaken. When treated by rapidly pronating and supinating the forearm the head of the radius relocates into the shallow depression on the lateral cortex of the ulna

  - ❏ There are no radiographic abnormalities with a nursemaid's elbow. The diagnosis is clinical. Radiography is not indicated.

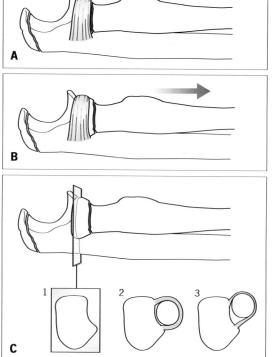

**Figure 5.6** *Pulled elbow / Nursemaid's Elbow. The usual theory is that the head of the radius subluxes distally under the annular ligament [A] and [B]. An ultrasound study[2] provides a different explanation [C]. A cross section at the level of the annular ligament demonstrates a shallow depression on the lateral margin of the ulna (1). The normal anatomy is shown in (2). A pulled elbow injury causes the head of the radius to perch on the anterior rim of the ulnar depression [3]. This ventral subluxation explains why a successful reduction is often preceded by a snap or a click which can be felt over the head of the radius; the click is caused by the head dropping back into its natural position alongside the ulnar groove.*

## STEP BY STEP ASSESSMENT OF THE RADIOGRAPHS

Most fractures around the elbow are readily identified (Fig. 5.7). The most common elbow fractures in adults involve the radial head or neck. The most common elbow fracture in children is a supracondylar fracture. Also, in children, fractures of the lateral condyle comprise approximately 20% of elbow fractures. If initial scrutiny does not show an obvious abnormality then the radiographs need to be re-examined using a precise and systematic approach.

■ In adults – *three questions to ask*

■ In children – *ask a fourth question*.

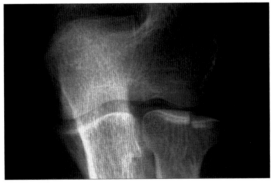

**Figure 5.7** *Fracture of the radial head. A common injury usually easy to detect.*

## ■ QUESTION 1

### Are the fat pads normal?

### FAT PADS

■ When a joint effusion is present it distends the capsule and displaces the fat pads away from the bone (Figs 5.5, 5.8)

■ A visible anterior fat pad is normal but if displaced anteriorly (the SAIL sign) it is abnormal

■ A visible posterior fat pad is always abnormal (Fig. 5.8). It denotes a large effusion

■ Not all joint effusions are associated with a fracture.[3] Nevertheless, in the context of trauma an effusion indicates that a significant injury has occurred even if a fracture is not seen

■ If there is displacement of either of these fat pads then the arm needs to be placed in a collar and cuff until an orthopaedic assessment occurs a few days later. This cautious approach recognises the fact that some of these patients will have an undisplaced fracture.[3–5]

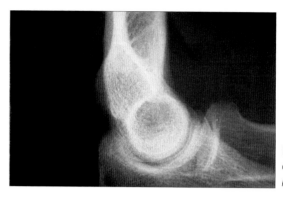

**Figure 5.8** *A large effusion displaces the anterior and posterior fat pads.*

---

**Pitfall:** Absence of a visible fat pad does not exclude a fracture. There are two possible explanations for this. The radial neck is usually extracapsular and thus a fracture of the neck may not produce a haemarthrosis and the fat pads will not be displaced. Alternatively, the joint capsule may rupture and the blood (haemarthrosis) drains from the joint.

---

## ■ QUESTION 2

### Is the radiocapitellar line normal?

**The rule:** a line drawn along the longitudinal axis of the radial head and neck should pass through the capitellum (Figs 5.2, 5.3, 5.9–5.11).

■ If this line does not pass through the capitellum then a dislocation of the radial head is probable

■ This rule is **always** valid on a true lateral film

■ Whenever there is a fracture of the shaft of the ulna the radiocapitellar line must be evaluated. There may be an associated dislocation of the radial head (Monteggia fracture dislocation). This Monteggia injury is particularly likely when there is angulation or displacement of the ulnar fracture (Fig. 5.11).

---

**Pitfall:** The radiocapitellar line can be affected by radiographic positioning. In children the rule is not always valid on the AP view because of eccentric ossification of the radial head or of the capitellar epiphysis. The radiocapitellar rule is best applied to a true lateral projection only.[6]

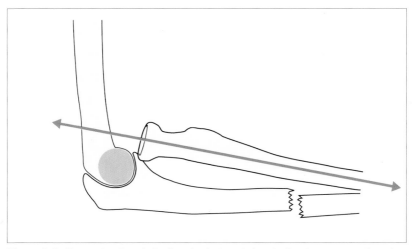

**Figure 5.9** *Abnormal radiocapitellar line. On the lateral view the line does not pass through the capitellum (shaded); this indicates that the head of the radius is dislocated.*

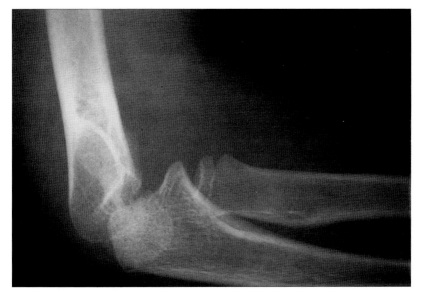

**Figure 5.10** *The radiocapitellar line does not pass through the capitellum. This indicates that the radial head is dislocated. Note: in this patient the abnormal alignment is the result of a dislocation of the entire elbow joint.*

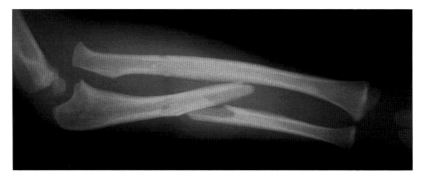

**Figure 5.11** *Fracture of the shaft of the ulna with over-riding of the fragments. The radiocapitellar line indicates that there is a dislocation of the radial head. This injury is known as a Monteggia fracture dislocation.*

## ■ QUESTION 3

### Is the anterior humeral line normal?

**The rule:** in most patients a line traced along the anterior cortex of the humerus will have at least one-third of the capitellum anterior to it (Fig. 5.4).

■ If less than one-third of the capitellum lies anterior to this line then there is the strong probability of a supracondylar fracture with the distal fragment (including the capitellum) displaced posteriorly (Figs 5.4, 5.12)

■ A supracondylar fracture is the commonest elbow fracture in children aged 4–8 years. It is a serious injury. Vascular damage, nerve injury, malunion or elbow deformity are potential complications. Evaluation of the anterior humeral line will prevent some of these difficult-to-see fractures from being overlooked.

**Pitfall:** This rule is not always reliable in very young children when there is only partial ossification of the capitellum. Nevertheless, if the anterior humeral line appears abnormal and a supracondylar fracture is not identified then the opinion of an experienced observer should be sought.

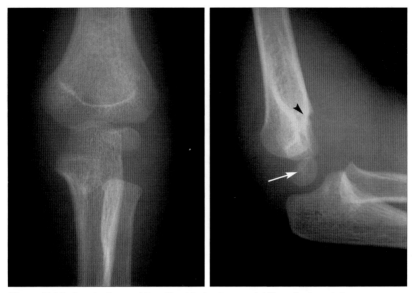

**Figure 5.12** *Anterior humeral line. The AP view is normal. When the lateral view was assessed it was noted that the anterior humeral line did not have a third of the capitellum (arrow) in front of it. This led to further evaluation of both the AP and lateral films and the supracondylar fracture (arrowhead) was identified. Note the displaced posterior fat pad.*

## ■ QUESTION 4: to be asked in all children

## Are the ossification centres normal?

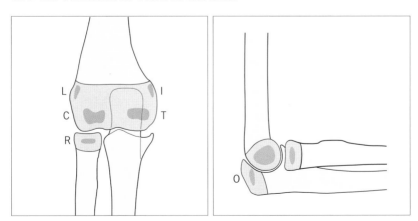

**Figure 5.13** *The normal ossification centres (dark shading) situated within the cartilaginous ends of the long bones. C = Capitellum; R = Head of radius; I = Internal epicondyle; T = Trochlea; O = Olecranon; L = Lateral epicondyle.*

■ At birth, the ends of the radius, ulna and humerus are present as lumps of cartilage that are not visible on a radiograph. The large empty gap between the distal humerus and the radius and ulna is normal

■ During childhood, six separate ossification centres (Fig. 5.13) appear at various intervals (6 months to 12 years). Four of these centres belong to the humerus, one to the radius and one to the ulna (Fig. 5.14). The four humeral centres gradually ossify, enlarge, coalesce and eventually fuse to the shaft

❏ The age at which each ossification centre appears is not important

❏ The order (Fig. 5.14) in which the centres ossify is important

❏ The acronym CRITOL gives the usual sequence in which the centres appear on the radiograph.

**Table 5.1** Elbow ossification centres

| Approximate age at appearance | Most common sequence |
|---|---|
| Birth ↓ 12 years | **C**apitellum<br>**R**adial head<br>**I**nternal (medial) epicondyle<br>**T**rochlea<br>**O**lecranon<br>**L**ateral (external) epicondyle |

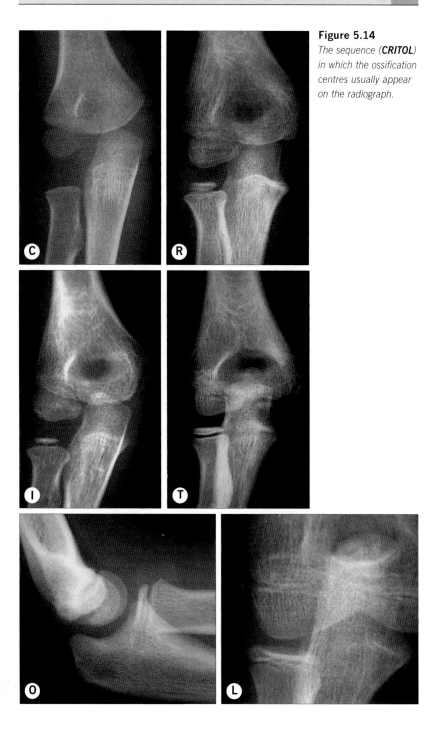

**Figure 5.14**
*The sequence (**CRITOL**) in which the ossification centres usually appear on the radiograph.*

## The importance of CRITOL

■ The ossification centre for the internal (i.e. medial) epicondyle is the point of attachment of the forearm flexor muscles. Vigorous muscle contraction may avulse this centre (Fig. 5.15). Avulsions are common in children who are involved in throwing sports. Hence the name 'little leaguer's elbow' given to this avulsion fracture. Paradoxically, minor displacement (Fig. 5.16) is radiographically more obvious than major displacement

■ When a major displacement of the internal epicondyle occurs the bone can become trapped within the elbow joint. This is a recognised complication of a dislocated elbow. In children, entrapment of the medial epicondyle after reduction of a dislocated elbow occurs in as many as 50% of cases.[7] The injury is easy to overlook when an elbow has been transiently dislocated and then reduces spontaneously.[7-10] When this occurs, the detached epicondyle may be misinterpreted on the AP radiograph as being the normal trochlear ossification centre (Fig. 5.17)

■ Though the CRITOL sequence does vary in normal children, the order is absolutely constant in one respect: the trochlear centre ossifies *after* the internal epicondyle. Thus, if the trochlear centre is seen there must be an ossified internal epicondyle visible somewhere on the radiograph. If it is not in its normal position then it could be trapped in the joint and masquerading as the trochlea

■ On occasion there will be uncertainty about the position of the internal epicondyle (or other ossification centres). Radiographs of the uninjured side can then be obtained in order to provide a comparison.

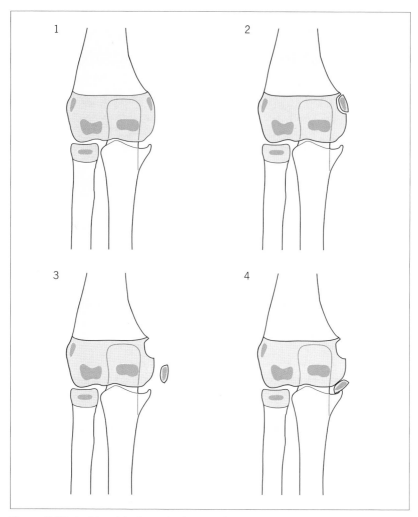

**Figure 5.15** *Avulsion of the internal epicondyle. 1 = normal; 2 = slight avulsion; 3 = major avulsion; 4 = major avulsion and the epicondyle lies within the joint.*

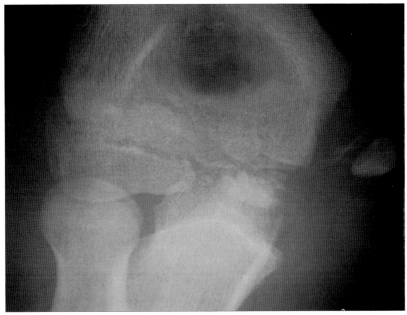

**Figure 5.16** *Avulsion fracture. Moderate displacement of the internal epicondyle.*

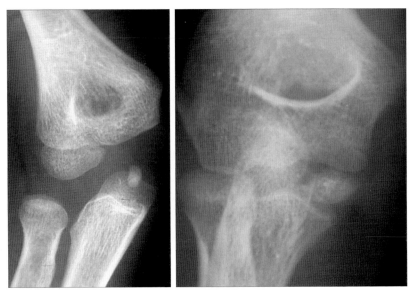

**Figure 5.17** *Two different patients. Major displacement of the internal epicondyle. In both patients the epicondyle lies within the joint.*

## PROBLEM: FAT PAD DISPLACEMENT
## BUT ... NO FRACTURE OR DISLOCATION IDENTIFIED

## THE NEXT STEPS:
### Adults

- No additional radiographs

- Treat as for a radial head fracture

- Clinical review in 10 days

  ❏ Clinically normal: no further radiography

  ❏ Clinically abnormal: obtain repeat views.

### Children

- It is most important that neither an undisplaced supracondylar fracture nor a displaced internal epicondyle is overlooked

- The radiographs need to be checked by an experienced observer before the patient is discharged from the Emergency Department. If a fracture is still not identified, then treat as for an undisplaced fracture

- Clinical review in 10 days

  ❏ Clinically normal: no further radiography

  ❏ Clinically abnormal: obtain repeat views.

## KEY POINTS

### FAT PADS

■ A visible anterior fat pad is normal. Displacement raises the possibility of a fracture

■ A visible posterior fat pad is always abnormal. Possibility of a fracture is increased

■ An undisplaced fat pad does not exclude a fracture.

### Radio-capitellar line

■ A line drawn along the long axis of the proximal radius should pass through the centre of the capitellum on the lateral film. If it does not – then a dislocated head of the radius is invariably present.

### Additionally, in children

■ Anterior humeral line. Normally, a third or more of the capitellum will lie anterior to this line. If it does not, suspect a supracondylar fracture

■ CRITOL is the most common sequence in which the secondary centres ossify. Though the precise CRITOL sequence will vary in some children there is one hard and fast rule: **'I before T'**. The trochlear centre does not ossify before the internal epicondyle. So, look for the **internal epicondyle**. If it is not identified – is it trapped in the joint and being mistaken for the trochlear ossification centre?

## THE SUBTLE SIGN NOT TO MISS

| Injury | Essential | Significance |
|---|---|---|
| Fracture of the shaft of the ulna. The radius is intact | Check the lateral view of the elbow Is the radiocapitellar (RC) line normal? Is the head of the radius dislocated? | An abnormal RC line indicates a Monteggia fracture-dislocation ❏ Often overlooked ❏ Delay in diagnosis puts a good outcome at risk ❏ Late complications include limitation of movement and deformity |

## REFERENCES

1. Greenspan A, Norman A. The radial head – capitellum view. Useful technique in elbow trauma. AJR 1982; 138: 1186–1188.
2. Berman L. Personal communication, 2004.
3. Donnelly LF, Klostermeier TT, Klosterman LA. Traumatic elbow effusions in pediatric patients: are occult fractures the rule? AJR 1998; 171: 243–245.
4. Griffith JF, Roebuck DJ, Cheng JC *et al.* Acute elbow trauma in children: spectrum of injury revealed by MR imaging not apparent on radiographs. AJR 2001; 176: 53–60.
5. Rogers LF, Malave S, White H, Tachdjian MO. Plastic bowing, torus and greenstick supracondylar fractures of the humerus: radiographic clues to obscure fractures of the elbow in children. Radiology 1978; 128: 145–150.
6. Miles KA, Finlay DBL. Disruption of the radiocapitellar line in the normal elbow. Injury 1989; 20: 365–367.
7. Chessare JW, Rogers LF, White H *et al.* Injuries of the medial epicondylar ossification center of the humerus. AJR 1977; 129: 49–55.
8. El-Khoury GY, Daniel WW, Kathol MH. Acute and chronic avulsive injuries. Radiol Clin North Am 1997; 35: 747–766.
9. Gore RM, Rogers LF, Bowerman J *et al.* Osseous manifestations of elbow stress associated with sports activities. AJR 1980; 134: 971–977.
10. Fowles JV, Slimane N, Kassab MT. Elbow dislocation with avulsion of the medial humeral epicondyle. J Bone Joint Surg 1990; 72B: 102–104.

# 6 WRIST AND DISTAL FOREARM

## ROUTINE

- PA
- Lateral
- Scaphoid series – when there is tenderness in the anatomical snuff box.

## ANATOMY

### POSTEROANTERIOR PROJECTION

#### Bones and joints

- The articular surface of the radius lies distal to that of the ulna in 90% of normal people (Figs 6.1, 6.2)
- The carpal bones (Figs 6.1, 6.2) are arranged in two rows. Strong ligaments bind the bones together
    - ❏ The joint spaces are uniform in width; 1–2 mm wide in the adult
    - ❏ Adjacent bones have parallel/congruous surfaces
    - ❏ Abnormally narrow spaces are probably due to radiographic projection or to degenerative change. Rarely due to injury
    - ❏ Abnormally wide spaces are likely to indicate an injury.

#### Soft tissues

The scaphoid (i.e. carpal navicular) fat stripe.[1,2] This is a thin layer of fat (black) that lies parallel to the radial surface of the scaphoid. Despite claims that effacement has relevance in trauma, this fat stripe can be ignored. See 'No longer a helpful hint' (p. 113).

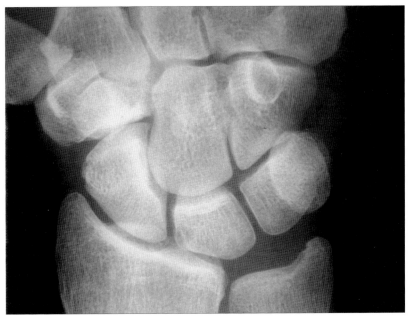

**Figure 6.1** *PA radiograph of a normal wrist. Note that the spaces between the carpal bones are uniform in size and that adjacent bone margins are parallel.*

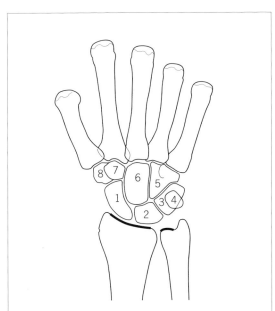

**Figure 6.2** *Normal wrist. The radial articular surface (dense line) lies distal to the ulnar surface in most people. A small notch on the lateral cortex of the radius is a normal variant even in adults – this is the site of the growth plate. The carpal bones: 1 = scaphoid (navicular); 2 = lunate; 3 = triquetral; 4 = pisiform; 5 = hamate; 6 = capitate; 7 = trapezoid (lesser multangular); 8 = trapezium (greater multangular).*

## LATERAL PROJECTION
### Bones and joints

■ The dorsal aspect of the distal radius is completely smooth – no crinkles, no irregularity

■ The alignment of the carpal bones may appear confusing but identifying the important anatomy is actually very simple (Fig. 6.3):

❑ The distal radius, the lunate and the capitate articulate with each other and lie in a straight line, like an apple in a cup sitting on a saucer (Fig. 6.4)

❑ The radius (the saucer) holds the lunate (the cup) and this cup contains the capitate (the apple)

■ The articular surface of the radius has a palmar tilt (Fig. 6.5). The angle of tilt is usually about 10° with a normal range of 2–20°.

### Soft tissues

The pronator quadratus fat line is a thin layer of fat (black) covering the ventral aspect of the pronator quadratus muscle. It is present on the radiographs of most normal adults.[1,2] Again, despite previous claims, displacement of this line is an unreliable indicator of injury. See 'No longer a helpful hint' (p. 113).

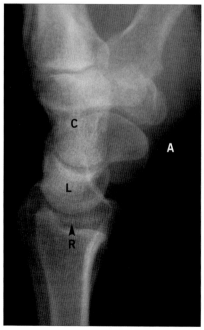

**Figure 6.3** *Lateral radiograph. Normal wrist. The important relationships are between the radius (R), the lunate (L) and the capitate (C). A = anterior.*

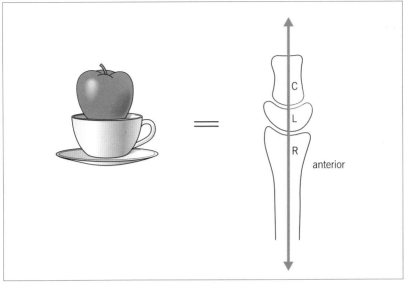

**Figure 6.4** *Lateral wrist. Normal. The radius, lunate and capitate lie in a straight line.*

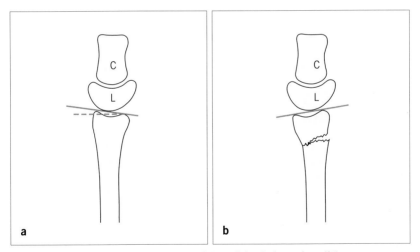

**Figure 6.5** *There is normally a palmar tilt of the radial articular surface. If the radiograph appears normal but palmar tilt is not present, suspect an impacted fracture. (a) Normal radius. (b) Fracture.*

## INJURIES

### FRACTURES[3,4]
### Distal radius
*Some are easy to recognise*

---

**Table 6.1** Easy-to-recognise fractures

---

**Posterior displacement distal fragment**
Colles'

**Anterior displacement distal fragment**
Smith's

**Children**

| Greenstick | Torus | Salter Harris II |
|---|---|---|

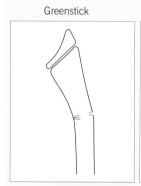 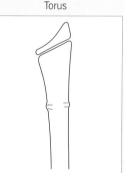 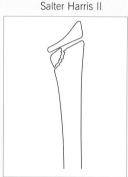

---

*Others are more difficult to recognise*

- A crinkle, or any irregularity of the cortex of the dorsal aspect of the distal radius (Fig. 6.6)

- An impacted and undisplaced fracture

  - ❏ The only abnormality may be a very slight increase in the density of the radial metaphysis (Fig. 6.7) and/or

  - ❏ Loss of the normal palmar tilt of the radial articular surface

- A longitudinal fracture extending to the joint surface

  - ❏ Frequently undisplaced (Fig. 6.8)

  - ❏ Some Barton-type fractures (Fig. 6.9)

- A slight ripple in the cortex visible in both projections, which represents a torus fracture (Fig. 6.10); a very common injury in young children.

# Wrist myths

- **No longer a Helpful Hint.** It is often claimed that if the pronator quadratus fat line is obliterated or irregular or shows anterior bowing, this raises the suspicion of an undisplaced fracture of the radius. An MRI study indicates that this much-quoted sign is completely unreliable.[5]

- Barton fractures are often incorrectly assumed to be any longitudinal fracture of the radius extending to the articular surface (Fig. 6.8). A Barton's fracture is a shearing fracture involving the distal radius and its articular surface. The fracture extends through the dorsal margin of the radius with the carpus following this distal fragment. A variation of this fracture (termed a reverse Barton's fracture or a volar Barton's fracture) is present when the anterior cortex is involved. Both types of Barton's fracture are important to recognise and categorise, as these are highly unstable injuries (Fig. 6.9).

- A beak or sharp lip of bone on the lateral aspect at the site of the fused growth plate is present in some adults. This is a normal appearance and should not be confused with a fracture (Fig. 6.11).

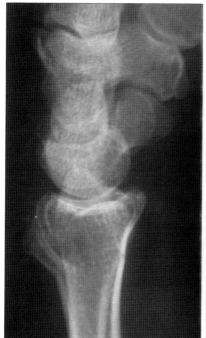

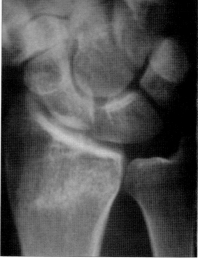

**Figure 6.6** *Fracture of the distal radius seen only on the lateral view. Also, note loss of the normal palmar tilt of the radial articular surface.*

**Figure 6.7** *An impacted undisplaced fracture of the distal radius is shown as a white (sclerotic) line.*

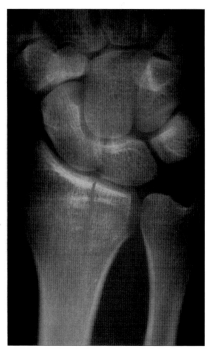

**Figure 6.8** *Undisplaced longitudinal fracture of the distal radius extending to the articular surface.*

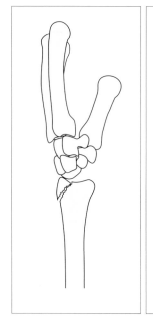 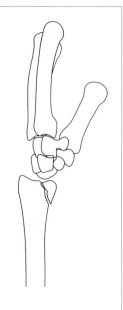

**Figure 6.9** *Barton-type fractures. On the left is a Barton's fracture; on the right is a volar (or reverse) Barton's fracture. These fractures involve the rim of the distal radius. Both fractures are unstable and frequently require internal fixation.*

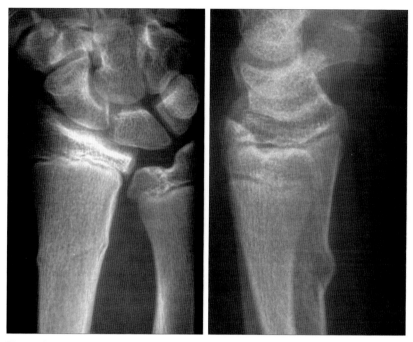

**Figure 6.10** *Torus fracture shown on both PA and lateral projections.*

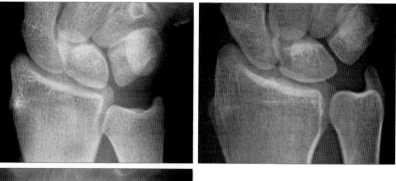

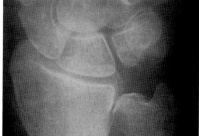

**Figure 6.11** *Pitfall.* A beak, or a small localized bulge of bone at the lateral margin of the fused epiphyseal line of the radius is a common normal variant. Three different patients.

## Scaphoid

■ A scaphoid series (not wrist views) should be requested when there is 'snuffbox' tenderness. The series comprises a standard set of four different projections (Figs 6.12, 6.13)

■ Fractures across the waist of the bone (Fig. 6.14) jeopardise the blood supply of the proximal fragment. If the patient is managed incorrectly then non-union, delayed union or avascular necrosis of the proximal fragment may result

■ If the scaphoid views appear normal it is mandatory that the patient is followed up. There are no exceptions to this rule (Fig. 6.15)

■ Some scaphoid fractures are not detectable until 5–10 days after the injury. By this time resorption of bone around the fracture has usually occurred and most fractures become obvious.

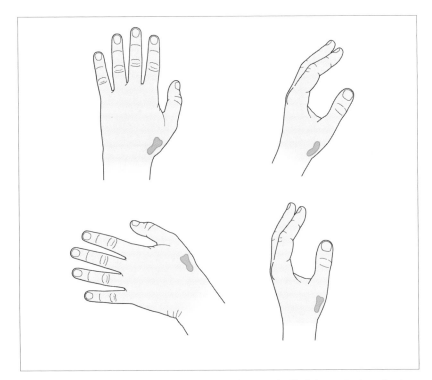

**Figure 6.12** *Scaphoid fractures are often very difficult to identify. It is standard practice to obtain four views.*

**Table 6.2** Risk of avascular necrosis in scaphoid fracture

| Site of fracture | Proportion of scaphoid fractures | Risk of avascular necrosis |
| --- | --- | --- |
| Waist | 80% | +++ |
| Proximal pole | 10% | ++++ |
| Distal pole | 10% | Nil |

**No longer a Helpful Hint.** If a fracture is not seen and the scaphoid fat stripe is bulging or obliterated it is often taught that an undisplaced fracture of the scaphoid is probably present. A MRI study has shown that this sign is unreliable and unhelpful.[5]

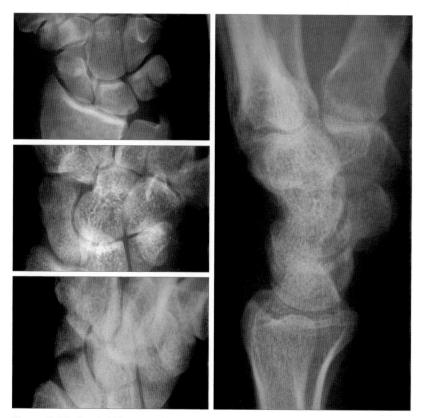

**Figure 6.13** *Scaphoid fracture – identified (with certainty) on one projection only.*

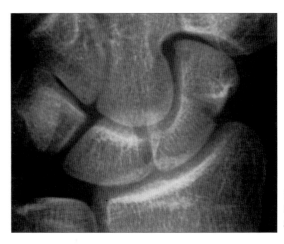

**Figure 6.14** *Fracture through the waist of the scaphoid.*

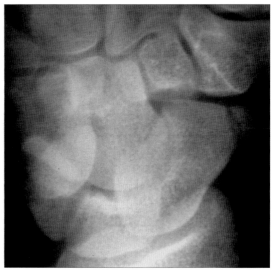

**Figure 6.15** *Fracture through the distal pole of the scaphoid.*

## Other carpal bones

- 95% of carpal bone fractures involve the scaphoid or the triquetrum. Fractures of the other bones are infrequent

- If a small fragment is seen lying posterior to the proximal row of the carpus on the lateral view, this invariably represents a fracture of the triquetrum (Fig. 6.16).

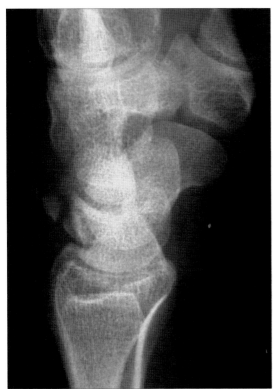

**Figure 6.16** *Two small bone fragments lie posterior to the carpus. Their origin cannot be clearly identified. Invariably, a fragment in this position represents a triquetral fracture.*

## SUBLUXATIONS AND DISLOCATIONS

### Distal radio-ulnar joint subluxation

- Common. Disruption of the radio-ulnar joint is a frequent finding with a Colles' fracture

- A fracture of the shaft of the radius with angulation or overriding and an intact ulna is invariably accompanied by separation of the distal radio-ulnar joint. This combination injury is termed a Galeazzi fracture-dislocation (Fig. 6.17).

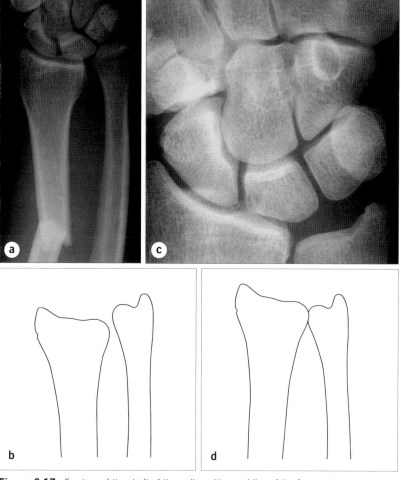

**Figure 6.17** *Fracture of the shaft of the radius with overriding of the fragments. The distal radio-ulnar joint is dislocated (a, b). This is a Galeazzi fracture-dislocation. Compare the appearance of the radio-ulnar joint in (a) and (b) with a normal wrist (c, d).*

## Lunate and perilunate dislocations[3,6,7]

Infrequent. These dislocations are not difficult to recognise provided that the normal anatomy on the lateral view is understood (Figs 6.3, 6.4).

**Normal anatomy:** the distal radius, the lunate and the capitate articulate with each other and lie in a straight line. The question to ask on all lateral views is 'does the capitate sit in the concavity of the lunate?'

*Lunate dislocation*

■ The lunate dislocates anteriorly. On the lateral view:

❏ *The concavity of the lunate is empty*

❏ The radius and the capitate remain in a straight line (Fig. 6.18)

■ Emphasis is often inappropriately placed on the appearance on the PA view because a dislocated lunate can adopt a triangular configuration (Fig. 6.18) instead of its normal 'squareish' contour (Fig. 6.17c). This sign can be helpful but it is much easier to diagnose the dislocation by assessing the lateral view.

*Perilunate dislocation*

■ A perilunate dislocation is often accompanied by a scaphoid fracture

■ The whole of the carpus (except for the lunate) is displaced posteriorly. Inspection of the lateral view will reveal the malalignment of the carpal bones (Fig. 6.19)

❏ *The concavity of the lunate is empty*

❏ The radius and the lunate remain in a straight line

❏ The capitate lies posteriorly and out of line.

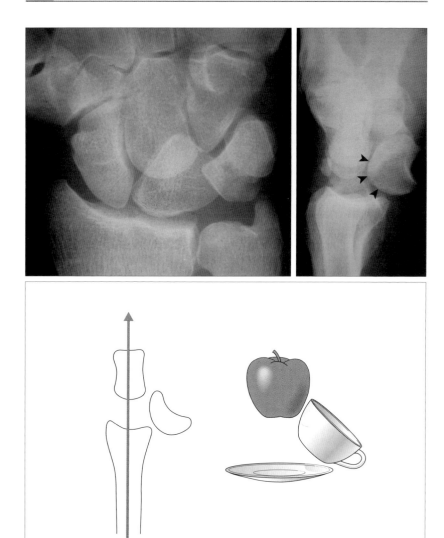

**Figure 6.18** *Lunate dislocation. The lateral radiograph shows the lunate (arrowheads) dislocated anteriorly. The concavity of the lunate ('the cup') is empty. The radius and capitate remain in a straight line.*

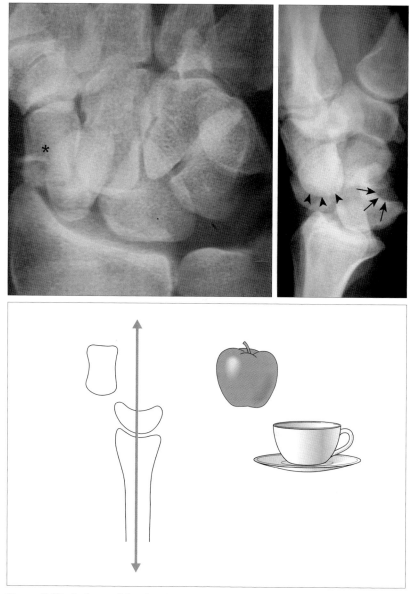

**Figure 6.19** *Perilunate dislocation. The concavity of the lunate is empty (arrows). The capitate (arrowheads) is displaced posteriorly. A scaphoid fracture (\*) is a common association.*

## Carpal subluxations[3,6,8]

- A ligamentous tear or rupture can affect any of the small joints of the carpus. This may result in carpal instability, pain, and reduced function

- Normally, the joint spaces between the intercarpal joints measure no more than 2 mm in the adult. Widening of any of these spaces raises the possibility of an intercarpal subluxation. In addition, subluxation will be suggested because adjacent bones do not have parallel or congruent surfaces. Referral to a hand surgeon for a specialist clinical evaluation will be necessary when joint widening or lack of parallelism is noted

- *Scapholunate dissociation is relatively common.* The scapholunate joint is particularly susceptible to ligamentous injury. An abnormal gap will be evident between the lunate and the scaphoid. This is sometimes referred to as the Terry Thomas or the Madonna sign* (Figs 6.20, 6.21).

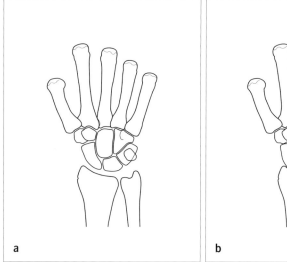
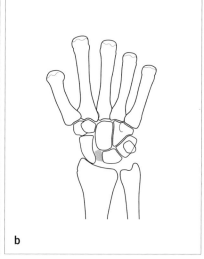

a    b

**Figure 6.20** *(a)* Normal PA view. *(b)* Widening of the joint space (shaded area) between the scaphoid and the lunate. This indicates an injury to the scapholunate ligaments.

---

* Terry Thomas was a 20th-century English comic actor, characteristically grinning and showing a trademark gap between the incisors. Madonna is a 21st-century actress and singer. An abnormal gap between the scaphoid and the lunate is therefore often called the Terry Thomas or the Madonna sign.

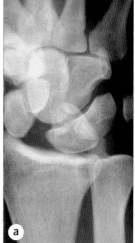
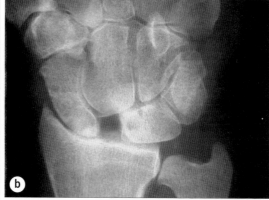
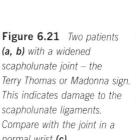
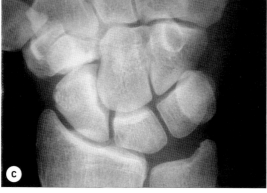

**Figure 6.21** *Two patients (a, b) with a widened scapholunate joint – the Terry Thomas or Madonna sign. This indicates damage to the scapholunate ligaments. Compare with the joint in a normal wrist (c).*

## COMBINATION INJURIES

■ Injuries to the wrist and carpus are not always solitary. They may occur as a mixture of the fractures and dislocations described above

■ The concept of a *zone of vulnerability* at the wrist is helpful in seeking for and identifying combination injuries

❏ The zone (Fig. 6.22) passes in an arc through the radial styloid process, the scaphoid, the proximal parts of the capitate and hamate, the triquetral and the ulnar styloid process

❏ If an abnormality is identified anywhere in this arc, it is essential to look for other fractures or dislocations across the zone (Fig. 6.19).

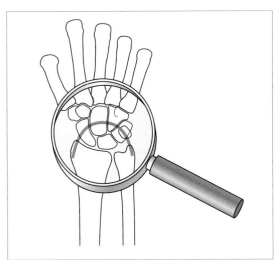

**Figure 6.22** *Zone of vulnerability (red arc). If one abnormality is detected within this area then it is important to look for another injury/ other injuries within the zone.*

## EVALUATING THE RADIOGRAPHS – A CHECKLIST

Many wrist injuries, diagnosed late, have an adverse effect on function.[8] When the radiographs appear normal it is useful to carry out a second search using a checklist. If an 'X' is placed in any of the boxes then the radiograph is abnormal and should be shown to an experienced observer.

**Table 6.3** Checklist for evaluation of wrist radiographs

| Clinical | Check that | ✔ = Normal<br>✘ = Abnormal |
|---|---|---|
| **Tender distal radius or proximal carpus** | 1. Palmar tilt of the articular surface of the radius is present | |
| | 2. The radial articular surface lies distal to the ulna | |
| | 3. The dorsal surface of the distal radius is smooth (i.e. no crinkle) | |
| | 4. The waist of the scaphoid is intact | |
| | 5. The capitate sits in the concavity of the lunate | |
| | 6. The intercarpal joints are no more than 2 mm wide and adjacent surfaces are parallel or congruous | |

## KEY POINTS

- Clinical examination determines the appropriate radiography: a wrist series or a scaphoid series

- A request for a scaphoid series means that the patient must be followed up – even if the radiographs appear normal

- The lateral projection may be the only view that shows a:
  - ❏ subtle ripple in the posterior cortex of the radius
  - ❏ torus fracture (see Particular paediatric points, p. 310)
  - ❏ triquetral fracture
  - ❏ dislocation involving the lunate

- The most common carpal dislocations (lunate or perilunate) are readily diagnosed from the lateral view. Apply the rule: 'the concavity of the lunate should never be empty'

- If an intercarpal joint measures more than 2 mm in an adult and/or adjacent surfaces are not congruous – suspect a ligamentous injury.

## TWO SUBTLE SIGNS NOT TO MISS

| Radiograph | Finding | Suspect |
|---|---|---|
| 1. Lateral | Reverse of normal palmar tilt of the articular surface of the radius | Impacted fracture of the distal radius |
| 2. Posteroanterior | Articular surface of the ulna lies distal to the articular surface of the radius | Disruption of the distal radio-ulnar joint, or impacted fracture of the distal radius |

# REFERENCES

1. Curtis DJ, Downey EF, Brower AC *et al*. Importance of soft-tissue evaluation in hand and wrist trauma: statistical evaluation. AJR 1984; 142: 781–788.
2. Zammit-Maempel I, Bisset RAL, Morris J, Forbes WStC. The value of soft tissue signs in wrist trauma. Clin Radiol 1988; 39: 664–668.
3. Goldfarb CA, Yin Y, Gilula LA *et al*. Wrist fractures: what the clinician wants to know. Radiology 2001; 219: 11–28.
4. Mayfield JK. Mechanism of carpal injuries. Clin Orthop 1980; 149: 45–54.
5. Annamalai G, Raby N. Scaphoid and pronator fat stripes are unreliable soft tissue signs in the detection of radiographically occult fractures. Clin Radiol 2003; 58: 798–800.
6. Curtis DJ. Injuries of the wrist: an approach to diagnosis. Radiol Clin North Am 1981; 19: 625–644.
7. Panting AL, Lamb DW, Noble J, Haws CS. Dislocations of the lunate with and without fractures of the scaphoid. J Bone Joint Surg 1984; 66B: 391–395.
8. Mayfield JK. Patterns of injury to carpal ligaments. Clin Orthop 1984; 157: 36–42.

# 7 HAND AND FINGERS

A basic knowledge of the anatomical attachments of the tendons and the ligaments is essential (Fig. 7.1) because a seemingly trivial fracture fragment can indicate that an important injury has occurred. Failure to recognise the relevance of a minor radiological finding may lead to inappropriate management and a significant and avoidable loss of function.

## BASIC RADIOGRAPHS

Clinical information indicating the precise site of injury will ensure that the most suitable radiographic projections are obtained.

| Injury | Radiographs |
|--------|-------------|
| Metacarpal or several phalanges | PA (Fig. 7.2) and oblique of the entire hand and wrist |
| Thumb or a single digit | PA and lateral of the thumb/digit only |

## ANATOMY

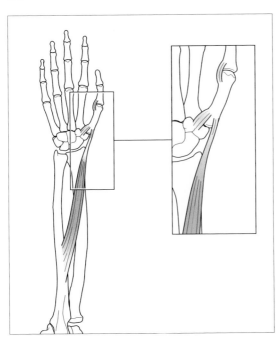

**Figure 7.1** *The thumb. Positions of some important muscle and ligamentous attachments. The insertion of the tendon of the abductor pollicis longus at the base of the first metacarpal; the medial ligament (i.e. the deep ulnar ligament) at the basal joint of the thumb; the medial collateral ligament at the metacarpophalangeal joint.*

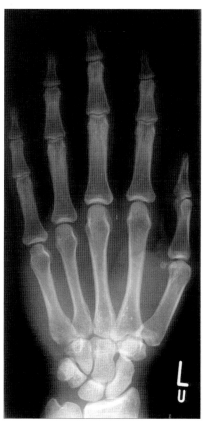

**Figure 7.2** *Normal hand. PA view.*
*Note that the joint spaces at the bases of the metacarpals are well seen and are the same width as the joint spaces between the carpal bones. The bones that articulate with the bases of the metacarpals are:*
*1 = hamate; 2 = capitate; 3 = trapezoid;*
*4 = trapezium. See magnified image below.*

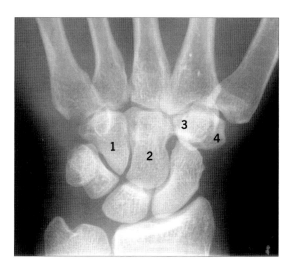

## FINGERS

■ The collateral ligaments extend from the lateral and medial margins of each metacarpal and each phalanx, across the joint, and insert into the same margin at the base of the adjacent phalanx (Fig. 7.3)

■ The extensor tendons insert into the dorsal surface at the base of each phalanx (Fig. 7.4)

■ The volar plate is a fibrous thickening of the joint capsule on the palmar aspect of each joint. It is attached to the base of the adjacent phalanx (Fig. 7.4)

■ At the bases of the fingers:

  ❑ The second and third metacarpals are attached to the carpus by thick, strong ligaments. The fourth and fifth metacarpals have fewer ligaments and are more mobile

  ❑ On the PA view of the hand (Fig. 7.2) the carpometacarpal joint spaces are clearly seen. They are equal (approximately 1–2 mm) in width

  ❑ The articular cortex at the base of each metacarpal parallels the articular surface of the adjacent carpal bone.

## THUMB

■ The stability of the carpometacarpal joint of the thumb depends on tough capsular ligaments.[1] The deep ulnar ligament is the thickened part of the capsule on the palmar aspect of the joint. This strong ligament extends from the first metacarpal to the trapezium (Fig. 7.1)

■ The tendon of the abductor pollicis longus is inserted into the radial aspect of the intra-articular portion of the base of the first metacarpal (Fig. 7.1).

---

**Pitfall:** The first carpometacarpal joint is very mobile. The amount of separation of the surfaces at the joint is variable and can be very wide. Normal variation may be mistaken for subluxation on a radiograph.

---

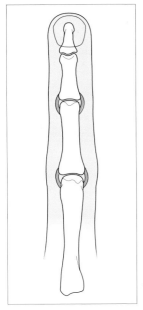

**Figure 7.3** *The medial and lateral collateral ligaments insert into the bases of the phalanges.*

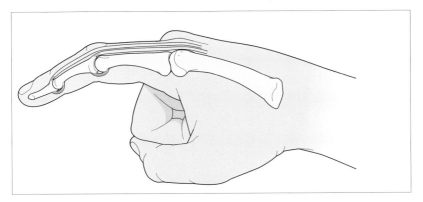

**Figure 7.4** *The extensor tendons (light shading) insert into the bases of the phalanges on the dorsal surface. The volar plate is a thickening (dark shading) of the joint capsule. It inserts into the base of the phalanx on its palmar surface.*

## INJURIES

## FRACTURES

### Hand and fingers

Most fractures involving the mid-shaft of a phalanx or of a metacarpal are stable. They pose few clinical problems. These phalangeal fractures are frequently managed by strapping to an adjacent digit (garter strapping or buddy strapping).

Some fractures will require careful orthopaedic assessment, particularly when there is:

■ Involvement of a joint surface (Fig. 7.5)

■ Avulsion of a fragment at the base of a phalanx (Table 7.1)

■ A flexion deformity (known as a mallet or baseball finger) of the distal phalanx. An isolated flexion deformity is almost impossible without either a rupture of the extensor tendon or an avulsion fracture (Fig. 7.6). Clinical examination is crucial since a fracture is present in only 25% of cases

■ A volar plate fracture, caused by forced extension of a finger. The detached fragment will be detected on the lateral view only (Fig. 7.7). These fractures are nearly always displaced and unstable

■ A fracture of a metacarpal neck:

  ❏ A fighter's (or scrapper's) fracture. When the blow is struck, the wrist is flexed. **Result:** fracture of the 4th or 5th metacarpal

  ❏ A boxer's fracture. Trained athletes strike with the wrist in the neutral position. **Result:** fracture of the 2nd or 3rd metacarpal

■ A spiral fracture of the shaft of a phalanx or metacarpal (Fig. 7.8) with rotation of the fragments. These fractures are often unstable and significant shortening may occur. Frequently require open reduction and internal fixation.[3]

**Table 7.1** Fingers: some small fractures are very important.

| Fracture fragment | Indicates avulsion of | Figure |
| --- | --- | --- |
| Lateral or medial | Collateral ligament | – |
| Dorsal | Extensor tendon | 7.6 |
| Palmar | Volar plate | 7.7 |

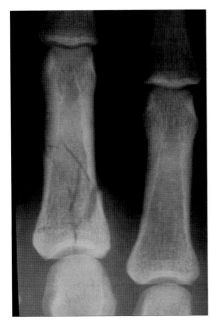

**Figure 7.5** *Undisplaced, intra-articular, comminuted fracture of the proximal phalanx. This injury is clinically important because the fracture involves the joint surface.*

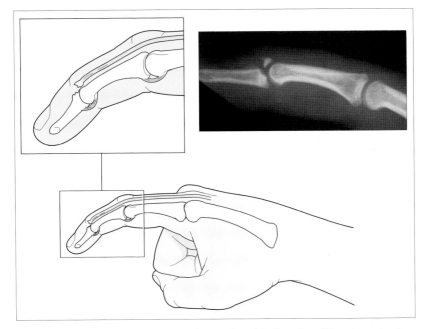

**Figure 7.6** *Fracture at the base of a phalanx at the point of insertion of the extensor tendon. This injury indicates a mallet (or baseball) finger.*

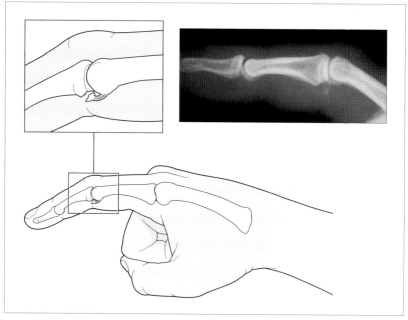

**Figure 7.7** *Fracture at the base of a phalanx at the point of insertion of the volar plate.*

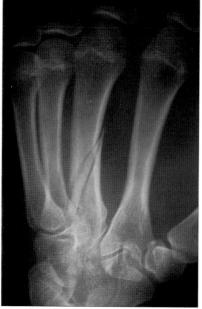

**Figure 7.8** *Spiral fracture of a metacarpal. The degree of rotation cannot be adequately assessed from the radiograph alone – clinical assessment is more accurate.*[3]

## Thumb

The basal joint (i.e. the carpometacarpal joint) of the thumb is multifunctional. It can adduct, abduct, oppose and circumduct. Injuries close to this joint need to be recognised, characterised and treated early.[1,2]

Distinguishing between an intra-articular and an extra-articular fracture at the base of the thumb (Figs 7.9, 7.10) is important. The distinction determines the appropriate treatment.

| **Table 7.2** Base of thumb fractures | | | |
|---|---|---|---|
| Intra-articular | = Bennett's fracture | = Unstable | Figs 7.9, 7.11 |
| Intra-articular | = Rolando's fracture | = Unstable | Fig. 7.12 |
| Extra-articular | | = Stable | Figs 7.10, 7.13 |

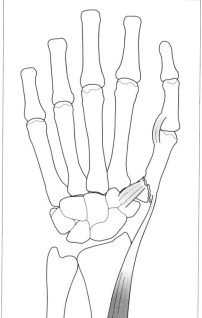

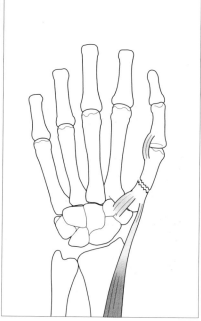

**Figure 7.9** *Bennett's fracture-dislocation. The intra-articular fracture involves the base of the first metacarpal. The larger metacarpal fragment is pulled dorsally and radially by the abductor pollicis longus muscle. An unstable injury.*

**Figure 7.10** *Base of thumb fracture. The fracture line is distal to the insertion of the tendon of the abductor pollicis longus. The carpometacarpal joint is not involved. No risk of dislocation.*

*Base of thumb: intra-articular fractures* (Fig. 7.9)

■ **Bennett's fracture.** A fracture involving the base of the first metacarpal (Fig. 7.11). This injury is more properly termed a **Bennett's fracture-dislocation.** See under Dislocations (page 140)

■ **Rolando's fracture.** A comminuted fracture of the base of the first metacarpal. The comminuted fragments often adopt a Y, V or T configuration (Fig. 7.12). Difficult to treat in terms of obtaining stability; frequently requires internal fixation.

*Base of thumb: extra-articular fractures* (Figs 7.10, 7.13)

The fracture line is distal to the joint capsule and distal to both the deep ulnar ligament and the insertion of the tendon of abductor pollicis longus. *There is no involvement of the carpometacarpal joint and no risk of dislocation.* Nearly all extra-articular fractures are treated by closed reduction.

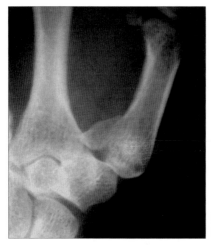

**Figure 7.11** *Intra-articular fracture. Bennett's fracture-dislocation – unstable.*

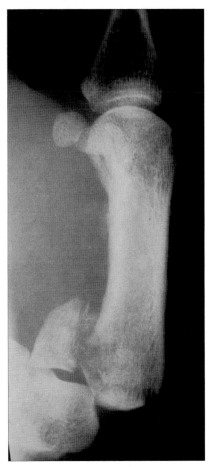

**Figure 7.12** *Comminuted intra-articular fracture base of first metacarpal. Rolando's fracture – highly unstable.*

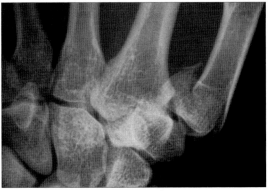

**Figure 7.13** *Extra-articular fracture at base of first metacarpal – stable.*

## DISLOCATIONS

### Fingers

Metacarpophalangeal and interphalangeal joint dislocations are easy to detect.

*Carpometacarpal joint dislocations*

- Occur infrequently.[3–5] They are clinically important and easy to overlook

- The fourth and fifth metacarpals are most commonly affected

- Dislocation is commonly associated with a fracture at the base of either the affected metacarpal or the adjacent metacarpal

- A fracture of the dorsal surface of the hamate (seen on the oblique view) should always raise the suspicion of an accompanying dislocation at the fifth carpometacarpal joint

- Effacement of a joint space at the base of a metacarpal on the PA view raises the strong possibility of this injury (Fig. 7.14)

- Lack of parallelism between the base of a metacarpal and the articular surface of the adjacent carpal bone is very suggestive of a dislocation.

### Thumb

- **Bennett's fracture-dislocation** is a common injury.[2,3] Early orthopaedic treatment (often open reduction) is essential because the multiple movements at the carpometacarpal joint are so important. The injury comprises a fracture at the base of the first metacarpal extending into the joint surface with dislocation at the carpometacarpal joint (Figs 7.9, 7.11). The larger metacarpal fragment is pulled dorsally and radially by contraction of the abductor pollicis longus muscle (Fig. 7.9). The deep ulnar ligament remains attached to the smaller fragment and the latter maintains its normal anatomical relationship with the trapezium. This is an unstable injury

- **Gamekeeper's/Skier's thumb.*** Rupture or severe stretching of the ulnar collateral ligament at the first metacarpophalangeal joint (Figs 7.15, 7.16)

  - Usually the ligament alone is torn and the radiographs appear normal. A complete tear of the ligament requires surgical repair[3,6]

  - Occasionally a bone fragment may be avulsed

  - Whenever there is clinical uncertainty as to the presence of a torn ligament, stress radiographs can assist in confirming or excluding the diagnosis.

---

* 'Gamekeeper's thumb' is due to chronic stretching of the ulnar collateral ligament. So called because of the method employed by 18th and 19th century English gamekeepers to break the necks of rabbits. 'Skier's thumb' occurs on the ski slope and is due to an acute tear of the same ligament.

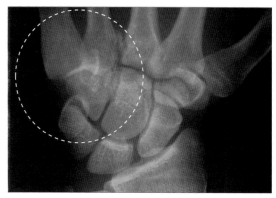

**Figure 7.14** *PA view. Carpometacarpal dislocation. The joint spaces at the bases of the fourth and fifth metacarpals are not visualised because the dislocated bones are overlapping.*

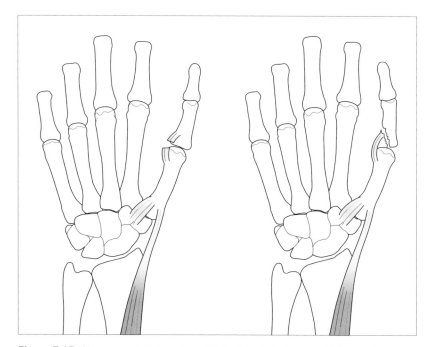

**Figure 7.15** *Skier's thumb. In most cases the medial collateral ligament is torn and the standard radiographs appear normal. Occasionally there is an avulsion fracture of the base of the proximal phalanx at the insertion of the ligament.*

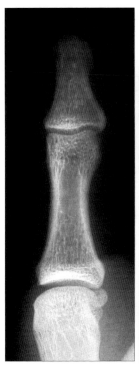

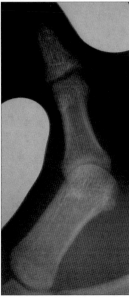

**Figure 7.16** *Right hand. Skier's thumb. The medial collateral ligament has ruptured. In the neutral position (left) no abnormality is apparent. When abduction stress is applied the excessive angulation at the metacarpo-phalangeal joint becomes obvious. No fracture. A normal sesamoid bone is present.*

## KEY POINTS

■ Small fragments of bone detached from the margin of a joint can have important functional implications and need careful orthopaedic assessment

■ A spiral fracture of a metacarpal with rotation of the fragments is an unstable injury and may require internal fixation

■ The key features of Bennett's fracture-dislocation:

  ❑ the fracture line involves the joint surface

  ❑ the medial fragment at the base of the 1st metacarpal maintains its relationship with the trapezium

  ❑ proximal and lateral subluxation of the metacarpal.

## THE SUBTLE SIGN NOT TO MISS

| Radiograph | Rule | If the rule is broken |
|---|---|---|
| PA of the hand | Each carpometacarpal joint should be well seen. The bones should not overlap | ■ Suspect a subluxation or dislocation at the carpometacarpal joint. Check the oblique view in order to exclude a dislocation |
| | | ■ Occasionally, the position in which the normal hand is held will cause spurious effacement of a joint |

## REFERENCES

1. Kauer JMG. Functional anatomy of the carpometacarpal joint of the thumb. Clin Orthop 1987; 220: 7–13.
2. Howard FM. Fractures of the basal joint of the thumb. Clin Orthop 1987; 220: 46–51.
3. Green DP, Rowland SA. Fractures and dislocations in the hand. In: Rockwood CA Jr, Green DP, eds. Fractures. Philadelphia: JB Lippincott, 1975.
4. Henderson JJ, Aarafa MAM. Carpometacarpal dislocation: an easily missed diagnosis. J Bone Joint Surg 1987; 69B: 212–214.
5. Mueller JJ. Carpometacarpal dislocations. Report of five cases and review of the literature. J Hand Surg 1986; 11A: 184–188.
6. Engkvist O, Balkfors B, Lindsjo U. Thumb injuries in downhill skiing. Int J Sports Med 1982; 3: 50–55.

# 8 CERVICAL SPINE

*Following trauma there is no need for radiography in patients who have no neurological deficit nor any neck pain or tenderness – as long as they are alert enough to say so.[1-5]*

## BASIC RADIOGRAPHS

■ Practice differs between centres.[6-9] Initial assessment is usually made with either a one-view, three-view or five-view trauma series

■ A three-view series is recommended. This should include:

  ❑ a lateral, which must show the top of the T1 vertebral body

  ❑ a long AP

  ❑ an open mouth AP to show the C1–C2 articulation – the peg view.

## ANATOMY

### NORMAL LATERAL VIEW
### Vertebral alignment

■ Three contour lines (or arcs) can be traced:

  ❑ Line 1: along the anterior margins of the vertebral bodies

  ❑ Line 2: along the posterior margins of the vertebral bodies

  ❑ Line 3: joining the bases of the spinous processes

■ These lines (Figs 8.1, 8.2) should be smooth, unbroken curves

■ Line 3 will sometimes show a slight step at the C2 level, particularly in children.[10] This step (Fig. 8.3) should not be more than 2 mm posterior to the smooth curve traced between C3 and C1.

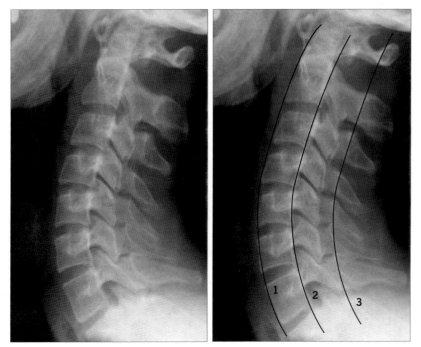

**Figure 8.1** *Normal lateral radiograph. The superior surface of the T1 vertebra must be included. The three smooth arcuate lines that need to be checked in all patients. The lines indicate whether vertebral alignment is normal.*

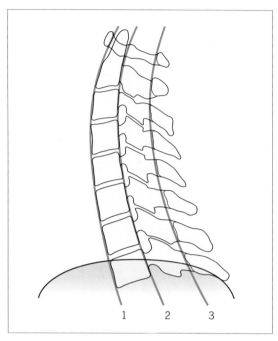

**Figure 8.2** *Normal lateral view. The three arcuate lines. Each line needs to be followed upwards and then downwards – this fail-safe checking ensures that a malalignment will not be missed.*

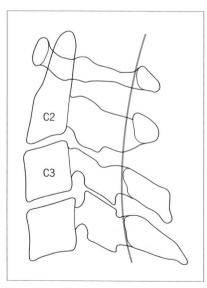

**Figure 8.3** *Alignment of the upper cervical vertebrae. When assessing the three arcuate lines, note that line 3 may not pass precisely along the base of the C2 spinous process. This is a normal finding provided that there is no more than a 2 mm gap between the C3–C1 line and the base of the C2 spinous process. Apply the rule: a gap larger than 2 mm is abnormal, and may indicate a fracture or dislocation at the C2 level.*

## Vertebral bodies

■ Those below C2 have a fairly uniform square or rectangular shape. The anterior and posterior heights of the vertebral bodies should be the same.

## Intervertebral disc spaces

■ These should be of uniform height.

---

**Pitfall:** Age-related changes occur. The development of osteophytes and the effects of disc degeneration can alter the anterior aspects/shape of the vertebral bodies.

---

## C2 vertebra and the odontoid peg (the dens)

■ Line 1 when continued superiorly merges with the anterior aspect of the peg

■ Line 2 when continued superiorly merges with the posterior aspect of the peg

■ On the lateral view the anterior arch of C1 appears as an oval or ring-like structure. The peg should be closely applied to this oval. The normal distance between the anterior aspect of the peg and the posterior aspect of C1 at this point is no more than 3 mm in adults and 5 mm in children (Figs 8.4, 8.5). The posterior aspect of the peg forms a continuous line (i.e. no step) with the posterior aspect of the body of C2 (Fig. 8.6)

■ Harris' ring of C2. The lateral view shows a white ring (Fig. 8.7) projected over the base of the peg and over part of the body of C2. This ring may appear slightly incomplete at its most inferior aspect (5–7 o'clock). This is a normal appearance. If any other part of the ring appears disrupted (see Figs 8.22, 8.24) then a fracture through the base of the peg needs to be excluded.[11]

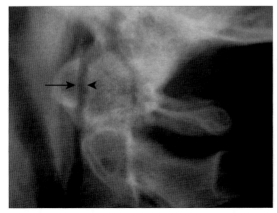

**Figure 8.4** *The normal distance between the anterior arch of C1 (arrow) and the anterior aspect of the odontoid peg (arrowhead) should be no more than 3 mm in an adult.*

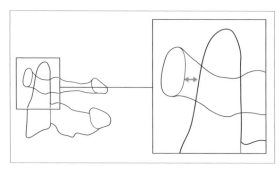

**Figure 8.5** *Normal relationship between the anterior arch of C1 and the odontoid peg. The distance indicated by the arrowheads should be no more than 3 mm in adults or 5 mm in children.*

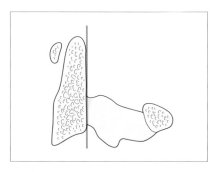

**Figure 8.6** *Normal anatomy. The posterior aspect of the odontoid peg forms a continuous line with the posterior aspect of the body of C2.*

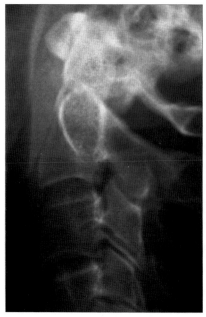

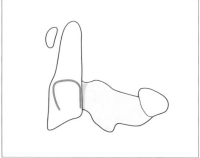

**Figure 8.7** *Harris' ring of the C2 vertebra. This ring is recognisable on most lateral views.[11] The normal ring is often incomplete in its inferior aspect.*

## Prevertebral soft tissues

- The soft tissue shadow[11–14] anterior to the vertebral bodies has a characteristic configuration (Fig. 8.8) and width (Table 8.1).

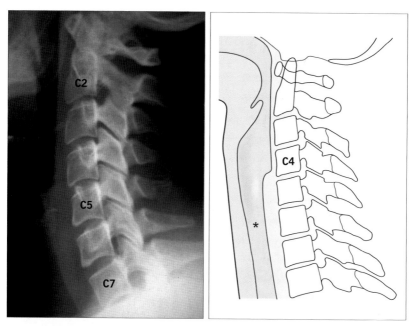

**Figure 8.8** *Normal width and configuration of the soft tissues lying immediately anterior to the vertebral bodies and posterior to the airway. C1–4 = 7 mm or less; C5–7 = 22 mm or less.* * = Trachea.

**Table 8.1** Maximum normal width of the prevertebral soft tissues

| Level | Width (mm) | Approximate % of vertebral body (AP) width |
|-------|-----------|--------------------------------------------|
| C1–4  | 7         | 30%                                         |
| C5–7  | 22        | 100%                                        |

## NORMAL LONG AP VIEW

■ The spinous processes lie in a straight line (Fig. 8.9)

> **Pitfall:** this rule may appear to be broken when bifid spinous processes are present (Fig. 8.10).

■ The distance between the spinous processes should be approximately equal. In normal patients no single space should be 50% wider than the one immediately above or below.[15]

> **Pitfall:** if the neck is held in flexion due to muscle spasm then this 50% rule will not apply.

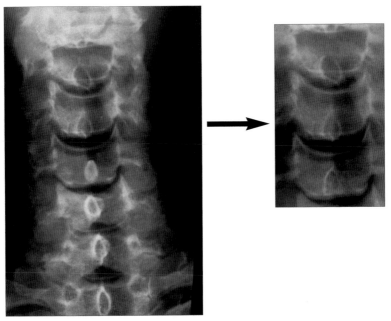

**Figure 8.9** *Normal long AP view. The spinous processes lie in a straight line. The distance between these processes should be approximately equal.*

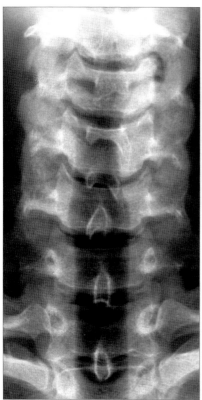

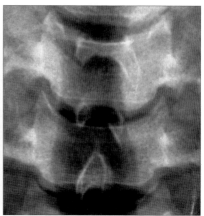

**Figure 8.10** *Spinous processes are commonly bifid. A bifid process may be asymmetrical. Sometimes this will incorrectly suggest that the processes are not in a straight line. The drawing shows a bifid spinous process as seen on the AP view and as it would appear if viewed from above.*

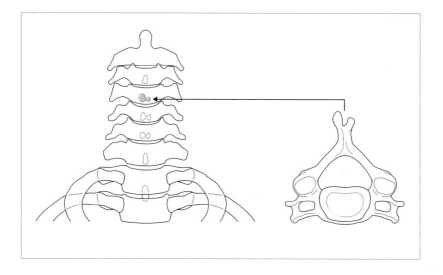

## NORMAL OPEN MOUTH AP – THE 'PEG VIEW'

■ The lateral margins of C1 should align with the lateral margins of C2

■ The distance between each side of the odontoid peg and the lateral mass of C2 should be equal (Fig. 8.11a).

**Caution:**

■ Slight rotation of the neck may cause these spaces to appear unequal. However, if the lateral margins of C1 and C2 remain normally aligned, then the asymmetry (Fig. 8.11b) can be attributed to rotation

■ Occasionally, asymmetry of the lateral masses of the vertebral body of either C1 or C2 (Fig. 8.12) will be present. This can mimic subluxation. Very often the explanation is slight rotation of the neck and/or developmental asymmetry of the lateral masses.[16–19] Occasionally, additional imaging is necessary in order to determine whether the appearance is a developmental variant or traumatic.

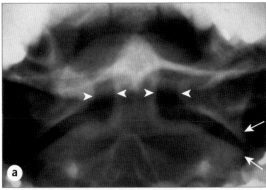
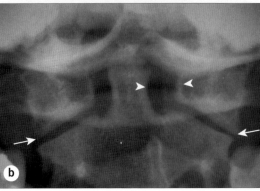

**Figure 8.11** *(a) Normal AP peg view. The odontoid peg is well seen and not obscured by overlying teeth. The space on either side of the peg is equal (arrowheads). The lateral margins of C1 and C2 align (arrows). (b) An apparent abnormality due to slight rotation of the patient's neck (see text). The space (arrowheads) to the left of the odontoid peg is wider than that on the right – but the lateral margins of C1 and C2 (arrows) remain in alignment. This confirms that the asymmetry is caused by slight rotation of the neck.*

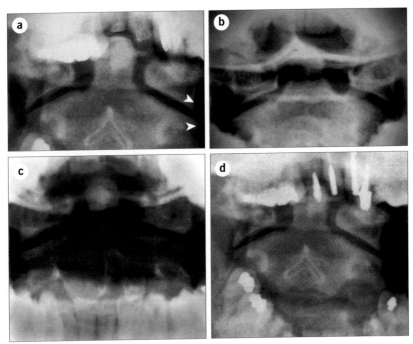

**Figure 8.12** Asymmetry at the articulations between the lateral masses of C1 and C2 vertebrae should be looked for. If present, it may indicate subluxation of one vertebra on the other. **Pitfall:** developmental asymmetry of a lateral mass does occur and can mimic subluxation.[16-19] Rotation of the neck is another cause of asymmetry. Examples: **(a)** The left lateral masses do not align (arrowheads). But all other margins line up. Also, the odontoid peg is not equidistant from each lateral mass. The asymmetry is due to rotation. **(b)** The margins of the lateral masses do not line up on the right side. But there is perfect alignment on the patient's left. Also, the odontoid peg is not equidistant from each lateral mass (wider space on the left). The asymmetry is due to rotation. **(c)** The right lateral masses do not line up on their medial margins. But all other margins do line up. Developmental asymmetry. **(d)** The left lateral masses do not line up on the far margin. But all other margins line up. A rotational effect.

## INJURIES

- 70% of detectable abnormalities will be visible on the lateral radiograph. Injuries are most common in the lower cervical spine (C5–C7) and at the C1–C2 articulation

- The radiographs must be inspected systematically. The following step by step approach is recommended.

## STEP 1: ASSESS THE LATERAL VIEW

### First, check that the top of T1 vertebra is seen

If the top of T1 is not demonstrated, then the radiographer must obtain further views (Figs 8.13, 8.14). There are several options: a higher-penetration technique, bringing the shoulders down by pulling on the arms, a 'swimmer's view' or trauma obliques.[8,9] Each of these additional views can be taken without moving the patient's head or neck.

### Secondly, trace the three contour lines or arcs (Fig. 8.15)

If there is a step or kink in any of these lines, suspect a fracture or ligamentous disruption.

---

**Pitfall:** The normal smooth cervical lordosis may be lost when the patient's neck is held in a hard or soft collar, or in spasm.

---

### Thirdly, check the vertebral bodies

- Below C2 these should be of a similar size and contour

- A detached fragment of bone may signify important ligamentous damage (Fig. 8.16)

- The spinous processes should be intact (Fig. 8.14).

### Fourthly, check the intervertebral disc spaces

Following a very severe injury, a disc space may occasionally be widened when compared with the other normal spaces above and below.[20]

## Finally, check the soft tissues

> *"An abnormal measurement or altered contour is usually due to a haematoma – this has a strong association with an important injury."*

■ Look for abnormal widening (Table 8.1), or a localised bulge (Fig. 8.17). Swelling of the prevertebral tissues occurs in approximately 50% of patients with a bone injury.[21] If soft tissue swelling is present then all the views need to be scrutinised again for other subtle evidence of a bone or ligamentous injury.

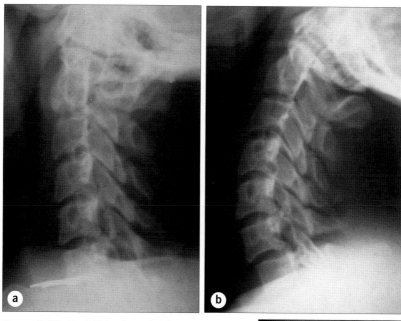

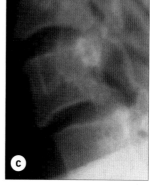

**Figure 8.13** *The initial radiograph* **(a)** *appears normal. But, C7 and the top of T1 vertebrae are not visualised. With the shoulders pulled down* **(b,c)** *the forward slip of C6 on C7 is revealed. Note: this film is still not adequate. Further views must be obtained in order to show the top of T1.*

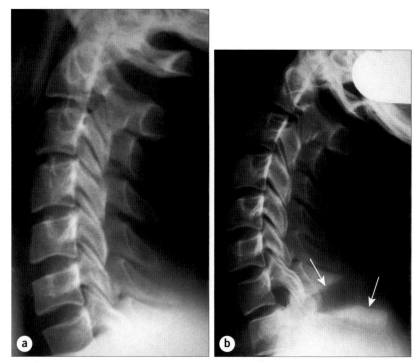

**Figure 8.14** *(a) No abnormality is seen. Patient discharged from the Emergency Department. But – the top of T1 vertebra has not been visualised. Patient recalled. The shoulders have now been pulled down (b). The repeat film (right) reveals a fracture of the spinous process of C7 (arrows) and anterior subluxation of the facets of C7 on T1.*

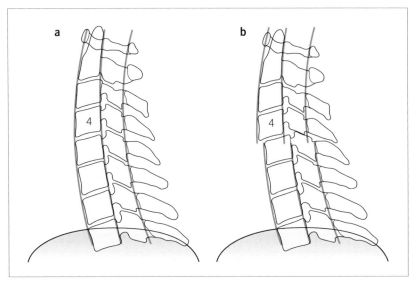

**Figure 8.15** *(a) The normal three smooth lines or arcs. (b) Disruption of each of the arcs, indicating anterior subluxation of C4 on C5.*

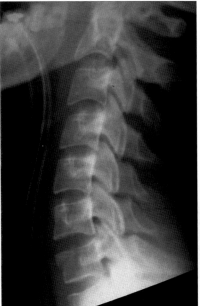

**Figure 8.16** *A small bone fragment is detached from the anterior aspect of C7. Although this may appear to be a minor injury it can be associated with major ligamentous rupture and instability. Note the endotracheal tube. Transection of the spinal cord was associated with this apparently trivial radiographic abnormality.*

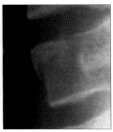

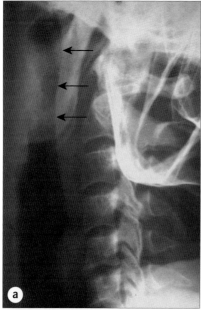

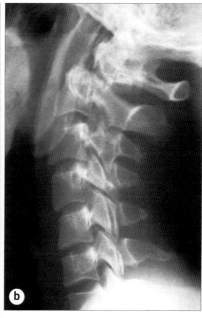

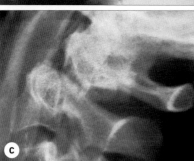

**Figure 8.17** *The importance of soft tissue swelling.* **(a)** *No bone injury was appreciated. Alignment, as indicated by the three arcuate lines, is normal. The only abnormality is extensive prevertebral soft tissue swelling (arrows). A repeat film 2 days later* **(b,c)** *shows a displaced fracture at the base of the odontoid peg with marked disruption of the three lines at the C1–C2 level.*

## STEP 2: ASSESS THE LONG AP VIEW

### First, check that the spinous processes are in a straight line

- If they are not in line − a unilateral facet joint dislocation must be excluded (Figs 8.18, 8.19)

- Whenever deviation of a spinous process is detected, the lateral view needs very careful reassessment.

**Note:** the spinous process of a vertebra as seen on the AP view is usually projected over the body of the vertebra at least one segment lower.

## Secondly, check that the distances between the tips of adjacent spinous processes are roughly equal

■ Abnormal widening of an interspinous distance (i.e. a space more than 50% wider than the space immediately above or below; Figs 8.20, 8.21) is diagnostic of an anterior cervical dislocation.[15] This observation is most useful in the severely injured patient whose shoulders have obscured some of the vertebrae on the lateral view[20]

■ Abnormal widening (page 160) provides an important warning that the neck must be managed very carefully whilst an adequate lateral view is obtained.

---

**Pitfall:** If the neck is held in flexion, abnormal widening may be due to projection only. Nevertheless, in the context of trauma, whenever this 50% rule is broken an injury should be assumed and an expert opinion obtained.

---

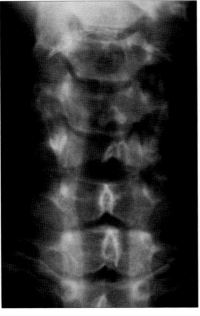

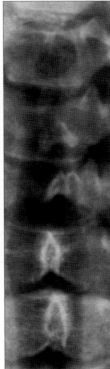

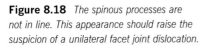

**Figure 8.18** *The spinous processes are not in line. This appearance should raise the suspicion of a unilateral facet joint dislocation.*

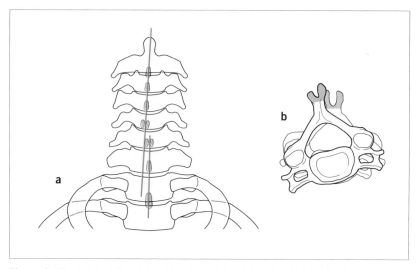

**Figure 8.19** *Unilateral facet joint dislocation.* **(a)** *A unilateral facet joint dislocation causes rotational displacement of adjacent vertebrae. The spinous processes do not lie in a straight line.* **(b)** *The displacement as seen from above.*

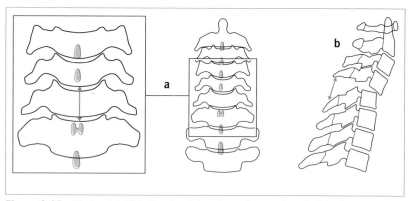

**Figure 8.20** *AP view.* **(a)** *Widening of an interspinous distance (arrow). This distance is 50% greater than the spaces immediately above and below.* **(b)** *When this finding[15] is present, it may well indicate an anterior cervical dislocation.*

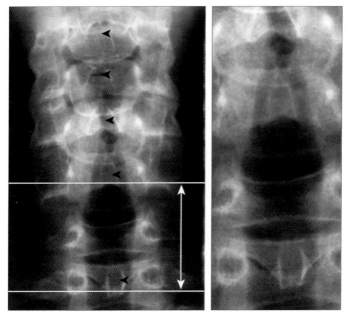

**Figure 8.21** *AP view. Abnormal widening of the space between the spinous processes (the two lower arrowheads). Assumption: a flexion injury with subluxation/dislocation.*

## STEP 3: ASSESS THE C1–C2 ARTICULATION

### On the lateral radiograph

Look for:

- A fracture of the odontoid peg (Fig. 8.17)
- Horizontal disruption (Fig. 8.22) of the Harris' ring of C2 vertebra
- Widening of the distance (Fig. 8.23) between the anterior margin of the peg and the posterior aspect of the arch of C1. It should be no more than 3 mm in an adult
- A fracture of the posterior arch of C1 or the lamina of C2 (Fig. 8.24)
- Displacement of the posterior arch of C1 from its expected alignment as part of the smooth curve of line 3 (Fig. 8.23)
- Prevertebral soft tissue swelling (Fig. 8.17).

## On the AP peg view

Look for:

- Fracture through the odontoid peg
- Displacement of the margin of either of the lateral masses of C1 away from the corresponding margin of C2 (Fig. 8.25)
- Unequal or increased spacing between the peg and the lateral masses of C2 (Figs 8.12, 8.25)

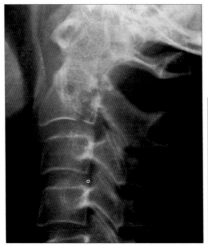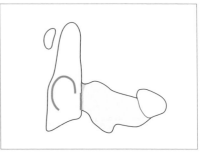

**Figure 8.22** *Fracture at the base of the odontoid peg extending into the inferior end plate of the C2 vertebral body. Note that the posterior white line of Harris' ring[11] is disrupted (drawing).*

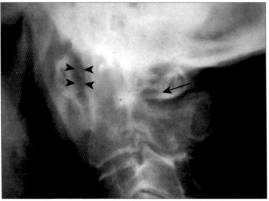

**Figure 8.23** *Adult. Abnormal widening of the space (arrowheads) between the odontoid peg and the anterior arch of C1 (normal = 3 mm) indicating anterior displacement of C1 on C2. Note: line 3 (the spinolaminar line) is also abnormal and the posterior arch of C1 (arrow) is displaced anteriorly.*

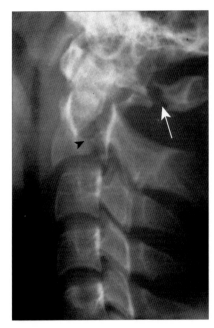

**Figure 8.24** *A fracture (a type of hangman's fracture) of the body of C2 (arrowhead). Also, fractures through the posterior arch of C1 (arrow).*

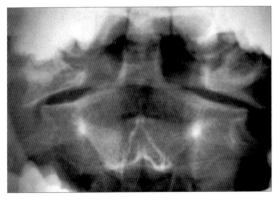

**Figure 8.25** *Burst fracture of C1 (Jefferson fracture). The space on each side of the odontoid peg is widened. The lateral margins of C1 overhang those of C2.*

## FOUR IMPORTANT PITFALLS

*Mach effect*

■ It is common to see a thin black line (Fig. 8.26) across the base of the peg that does not represent a fracture. The optical illusion results from overlapping shadows from superimposed structures. It is known as a Mach band or Mach effect.[22] It is important to be aware of these lines. It is even more important to seek advice before too readily dismissing any line as an artefact.

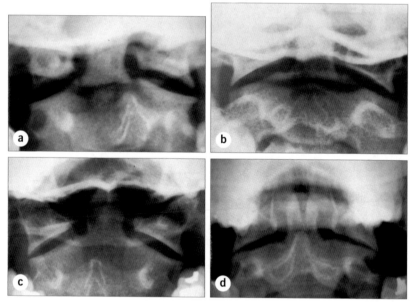

**Figure 8.26** *Pitfalls: common artefacts on the open mouth AP peg view.*
*Spurious appearances mimicking fractures due to Mach bands:* **(a, b)** *at the base of the odontoid peg;* **(c)** *at the tip of the peg. The superimosed structure causing these Mach effects is variable: the back of the tongue, the posterior or anterior arch of C1, the occiput, the lips or a neck skin crease. The appearance of a vertical split of the peg* **(d)** *is due to overlap with the upper incisor teeth.*

*Developmental variants*

- A vertebra might appear slightly narrow anteriorly with loss of the normal square or rectangular outline (Fig. 8.27). This can mimic a compression fracture. Although this narrowing is sometimes due to old trauma or aging it is often due to persistence of the normal, slightly wedge shape that is present during adolescence[23]

- A small calcified opacity anterior to a vertebral body (Fig. 8.27) can be mistaken for a fracture fragment. Sometimes this represents a detached osteophyte from a previous injury. Alternatively, it might be a remnant of an ununited secondary ossification centre.[23] When such an opacity is detected, an experienced observer should review the radiographs.

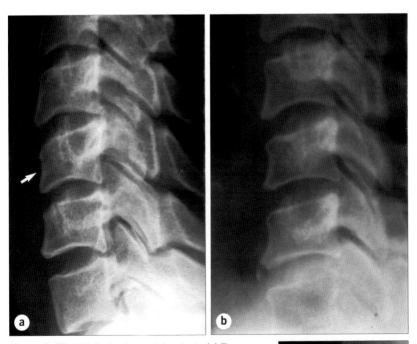

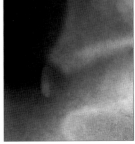

**Figure 8.27** *Pitfall: developmental variants.* **(a)** *The anterior aspect of a vertebral body (arrow) may appear slightly flattened. In this instance it is due to persistence of the normal wedge-shaped configuration commonly present during adolescence. Distinguishing this appearance from a fracture may be difficult.* **(b)** *Calcification close to the anterior longitudinal ligament may mimic a fracture fragment. This is often due to a persistent unfused secondary ossification centre belonging to the adjacent vertebral body. An age-related osteophyte can also produce a similar appearance.*

*Cervical spondylosis*

- Degenerative changes are common over the age of 40. Distinguishing between changes due to spondylosis and those resulting from an acute injury is not always easy. The following are frequently present in the middle-aged and elderly

  - The anterior margin of a vertebral body shows a step on the vertebra below (Fig. 8.28). This is due to an osteophyte. It may be misinterpreted as indicating vertebral subluxation

  - Anterior subluxation (Fig. 8.29) secondary to facet joint osteoarthritis. There is no simple way of distinguishing this from traumatic subluxation on the plain radiographs

- Fortunately, correlation of the clinical symptoms and signs with the site of the radiographic abnormality will provide reassurance in most instances. In other cases an injury should be assumed until an experienced observer has reviewed the radiographs.[24]

*Delayed instability*

- Severe pain and spasm may make it difficult to exclude a significant injury to the posterior ligament complex. Muscle spasm can hold the neck in an anatomical position and mask ligamentous rupture. Instability may only become evident after a few days when the spasm has resolved. For this reason it is important that any patient who has severe pain and spasm but appears fit for discharge is put in a collar and asked to re-attend within a few days for lateral views in flexion and extension. These radiographs must be taken under close clinical supervision.

  If the additional plain film findings remain equivocal, it will usually be necessary to refer the patient for MRI to exclude a ligamentous injury.

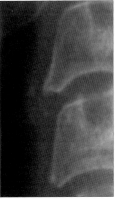

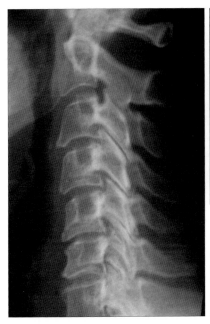

**Figure 8.28** *Pitfall: degenerative change.*
A step may occur in the smooth arc (line 1)
that extends along the anterior margin of the
vertebral bodies. In this patient the step is due
to anterior osteophyte formation at the inferior
margin of C3.

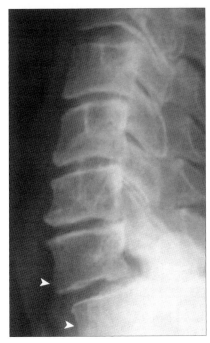

**Figure 8.29** *Pitfall: degenerative
change.* Forward subluxation of the
body of C7 on T1 is secondary to facet
joint osteoarthritis. This appearance is
radiologically indistinguishable from a
traumatic subluxation.

## KEY POINTS

■ The majority of injuries are shown on the lateral radiograph

■ The following need to be checked:

On the *lateral view*
❏ top of T1 visible
❏ three smooth arcs maintained
❏ vertebral bodies of uniform height
❏ odontoid peg intact and closely applied to C1
❏ no localised bulge in the prevertebral soft tissues

On the *long AP view*
❏ spinous processes in a straight line and spaced equally

On the *open mouth AP peg view*
❏ peg intact
❏ equal spaces on either side of the peg
❏ lateral margins of C1 and C2 align

■ *Be cautious.* An important neck injury may still be present despite normal plain films. Clinical history and examination must always take precedence over apparently normal radiographs.

## THE SUBTLE SIGN NOT TO MISS

| Radiographic projection | The sign to look for | Indicates | Described on page |
|---|---|---|---|
| Lateral | A horizontal break in the white ring of C2 | A low fracture of the odontoid peg[11] | 147 |

## REFERENCES

1. Clancy MJ. Clearing the cervical spine of adult victims of trauma. J Accid Emerg Med 1999; 16: 208–214.
2. Frohna WJ. Emergency Department evaluation and treatment of the neck and cervical spine injuries. Emerg Med Clin North Am 1999; 17: 739–790.
3. Stiell IG, Wells GA et al. The Canadian C-spine rule for radiography in alert and stable trauma patients. JAMA 2001; 286: 1841–1848.

4. Ivy ME, Cohn SM. Addressing the myths of cervical spine injury management. Am J Emerg Med 1997; 15: 591–595.

5. Brohi K, Wilson-Macdonald J. Evaluation of unstable cervical spine injury: a 6-year experience. J Trauma 2000; 49: 76–80.

6. West OC, Anbari MM, Pilgram TK et al. Acute cervical spine trauma: diagnostic performance of single-view versus three-view radiographic screening. Radiology 1997; 204: 819–823.

7. Marx JA, Biros MH. Who is at low risk after head or neck trauma? N Engl J Med 2000; 343: 137–140.

8. MacDonald RL, Schwartz ML, Mirich D et al. Diagnosis of cervical spine injury in motor vehicle crash victims: how many X-rays are enough? J Trauma 1999; 30: 392–397.

9. Turetsky DB, Vines FS, Clayman DA, Northup HM. Technique and use of supine oblique views in acute cervical spine trauma. Ann Emerg Med 1993; 22: 685–689.

10. Harris JH, Mirvis SE. The radiology of acute cervical spine trauma, 3rd ed. Baltimore, MD: Williams & Wilkins; 1996: 16–20.

11. Harris JH, Burke JT, Ray DD et al. Low (type III) odontoid fractures: a new radiographic sign. Radiology 1984; 153: 353–356.

12. Harris JH. The cervicocranium: its radiographic assessment. Radiology 2001; 218: 337–381.

13. Herr CH, Ball PA, Sargent SK et al. Sensitivity of prevertebral soft tissue measurement at C3 for detection of cervical spine fractures and dislocations. Am J Emerg Med 1998; 16: 346–349.

14. Matar LD, Doyle AJ. Prevertebral soft-tissue measurements in cervical spine injury. Austr Radiol 1997; 41: 229–237.

15. Naidich JB, Naidich TP, Garfein C et al. The widened interspinous distance: a useful sign of anterior cervical dislocation in the supine frontal projection. Radiology 1977; 123: 113–116.

16. Gehweiler JA Jr, Daffner RH, Roberts L Jr. Malformations of the atlas vertebra simulating the Jefferson fracture. AJR 1983; 140: 1083–1086.

17. Suss RA, Zimmerman RD, Leeds NE. Pseudospread of the atlas: false sign of Jefferson fracture in young children. AJR 1983; 140: 1079–1082.

18. Barton D, Redmond HP, Quinlan W. Radiological assessment of atlanto-axial injuries. Injury 1989; 20: 42–45.

19. Mirvis SE. How much lateral atlantodental interval asymmetry and atlantoaxial lateral mass asymmetry is acceptable on an open-mouth odontoid radiograph, and when is additional investigation necessary? AJR 1998; 170: 1106–1107.

20. Harris JH, Yeakley JS. Radiographically subtle soft tissue injuries of the cervical spine. Curr Prob Diagn Radiol 1989; 18: 161–192.

21. Miles KA, Finlay D. Is prevertebral soft tissue swelling a useful sign in injury of the cervical spine? Injury 1988; 19: 177–179.

22. Daffner RH. Pseudofracture of the dens: Mach bands. AJR 1977; 128: 607–612.

23. Keats TE. Atlas of normal Roentgen variants that may simulate disease, 7th edn. Chicago, IL: Year Book; 2001.

24. Lee C, Woodring JH, Rogers LF et al. The radiographic distinction of degenerative slippage (spondylolisthesis and retrolisthesis) from traumatic slippage of the cervical spine. Skeletal Radiol 1986; 15: 439–443.

# 9 THORACIC AND LUMBAR SPINE

Whenever plain radiographs are obtained the three column principle should be applied (Fig. 9.1).[1–3]

*"Instability is present if any two of the three columns are disrupted"*

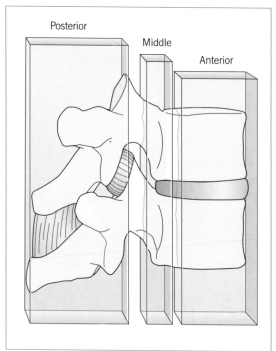

**Figure 9.1** *The three column spine. Assessment of each column is important. Note the normal concavity of the posterior margin of the vertebral bodies.*

**Table 9.1** The three column spine

| Column | Components |
|---|---|
| Anterior | The anterior longitudinal ligament, the anterior part of the annulus fibrosus, and the anterior two thirds of the vertebral body |
| Middle | The posterior longitudinal ligament, the posterior part of the annulus fibrosus, and the posterior margin of the vertebral body |
| Posterior | The posterior bone arch and the posterior ligaments |

## BASIC RADIOGRAPHS

■ Lateral

■ AP.

## ANATOMY

### LATERAL PROJECTION

■ The contour of the lumbar spine is a smooth unbroken arc (Fig. 9.2)

■ The vertebral bodies are the same height anteriorly and posteriorly (Fig. 9.2)

■ The posterior margin of each vertebral body is slightly concave (Figs 9.1 and 9.2)

■ Each of the three columns is normal – i.e. no step, break or kink (Figs 9.1, 9.2).

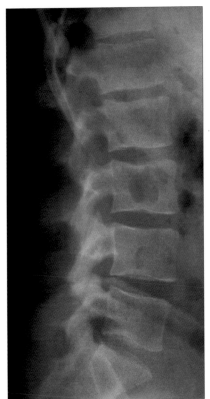

**Figure 9.2** *Normal lumbar spine. The anterior and posterior margins of the vertebral bodies form smooth arcs – no step or kink. The posterior margins of the vertebral bodies are concave.*

## AP PROJECTION

■ In the thoracic spine the soft tissue shadow of the left paraspinal line (Figs 9.3, 9.4) should be closely applied to the vertebral bodies. This line is produced by the interface between the paravertebral soft tissues and the adjacent lung. On the right side there is no paraspinal line[4,5]

■ In the lumbar spine there is no paraspinal line

■ In the lumbar region the distance between the pedicles (Fig. 9.5) should become gradually wider apart when descending from L1 to L5.

> **Pitfall:** The thoracic right paraspinal line may appear in the middle-aged and elderly when the pleura is displaced by age-related lateral osteophytes.

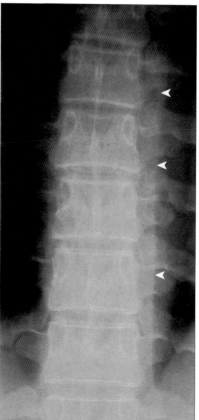

**Figure 9.3** *Normal thoracic spine. The left paraspinal line (arrowheads) parallels the lateral margin of the vertebral bodies.*

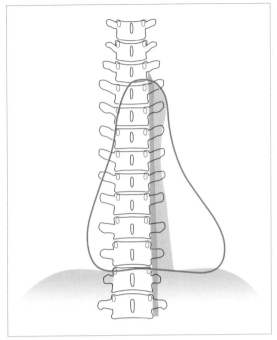

**Figure 9.4** *The normal paraspinal line (blue shading) is seen adjacent to the left lateral margin of the vertebral bodies. The brown shading further laterally is the normal descending aorta.*

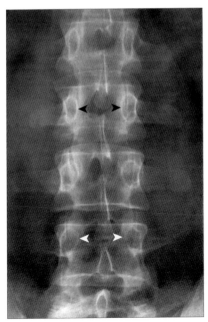

**Figure 9.5** *Normal lumbar vertebrae. The pedicles become slightly wider apart when progressing from L1 to L5. For example, the pedicles of L4 (white arrowheads) are slightly wider apart than those of L2 (black arrowheads).*

- Some patients with a severe fracture may not demonstrate any neurological abnormality. Symptoms and signs are often delayed

- 70–90% of detectable plain film abnormalities will be shown on the lateral projection[6,7]

- The clinical significance of a wedge fracture may be underestimated. These fractures (Fig. 9.7) can cause middle column bone fragments to intrude into the spinal canal.

## ON THE LATERAL VIEW

Look for:

- Loss of height or wedging of a vertebral body: this is evidence of a compression fracture (Fig. 9.6). Wedging may be associated with loss of the normal concavity of the posterior aspect of the vertebral body.[8] This indicates significant posterior displacement of the middle column (Fig. 9.7)

- Fragment(s) of bone detached from the anterior aspect of a vertebral body (Figs 9.6, 9.7, 9.8)

- More than one abnormality. The importance of recognising all abnormalities is explained under Stability, below.

## ON THE AP VIEW

Look for:

- Localised displacement or widening of the thoracic paraspinal lines (Figs 9.9, 9.10). In the context of trauma, this should be regarded as indicating a paraspinal haematoma resulting from a fracture

- Abnormal widening of the distance between the pedicles (Fig. 9.11). This indicates that fracture fragments have splayed apart

- A fracture of a transverse process. These can be subtle; a bright light or windowing on digital images will usually be necessary.

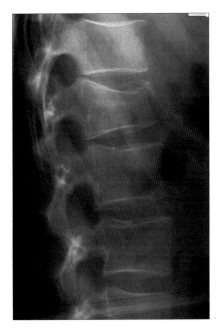

**Figure 9.6** *Wedge compression fracture of L1. The normal posterior concavity of the vertebral body is preserved.*

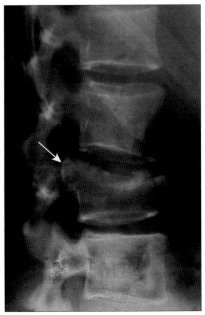

**Figure 9.7** *This patient had fallen from a horse 3 days previously and, despite back pain, had been able to continue at work. Wedge fracture of L3 vertebral body; its normal posterior concavity is lost. Two of the three columns are disrupted and this is an unstable fracture. Bone fragments (arrow) have been displaced into the spinal canal.*

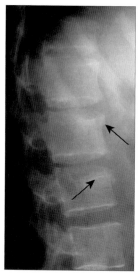

**Figure 9.8** *Wedge compression fractures of the L2 and L3 vertebral bodies (arrows). There is also a compression fracture of the body of T12.*

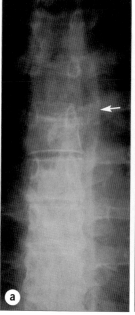

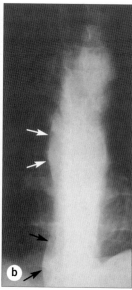

**Figure 9.9** *Abnormal paraspinal lines – two different patients. Each had fallen and complained of thoracic pain.* **(a)** *A haematoma produces a left-sided bulge (arrow).* **(b)** *Two separate haematomas produce right-sided bulges. These abnormal soft tissue appearances (arrowed) were associated with adjacent vertebral body fractures.*

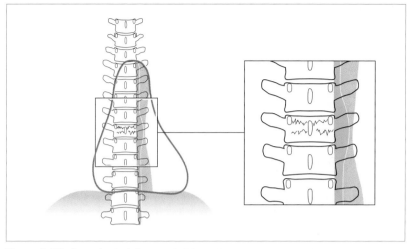

**Figure 9.10** *Example: the left paraspinal line bulges laterally in the mid-thoracic region. This is due to the haematoma around the fracture of T8 vertebral body.*

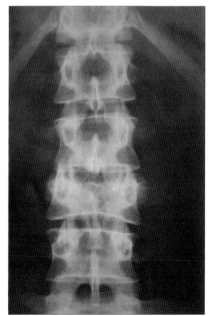

**Figure 9.11** *A wider distance between the pedicles of L3 when compared with the interpediculate distance of the vertebral body below. This is the reverse of normal, and indicates a fracture of L3 vertebral body.*

## STABILITY

- When an abnormality is detected it needs to be categorised as stable or unstable

- The concept of three columns[3] is a familiar one when evaluating a CT or MRI examination. The concept can also be applied to the plain radiographs. This approach to evaluating the plain films may provide an early indication, when signs and symptoms are minimal, that a potentially catastrophic injury is present

- Instability is present if any two of the three columns are disrupted (Figs 9.7, 9.12)

- The term 'stable injury' should only be applied to minimal/moderate compression fractures with an intact posterior column.[3]

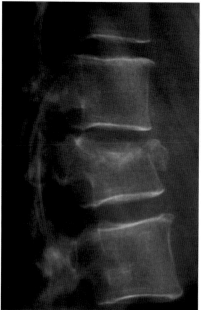

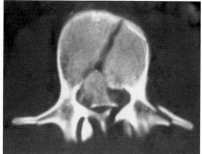

**Figure 9.12** *Fracture of the body of L1. The plain film shows disruption of two of the three columns. An unstable injury. Computed tomography shows that all three columns are disrupted. A large fragment from the posterior column lies in the spinal canal. Fractures of the transverse processes are also present.*

## KEY POINTS

- Some serious injuries are not always clinically obvious. The plain radiographs may indicate that severe trauma has occurred
- The lateral projection gives most information. Check that:
  - ❏ the vertebral bodies are of equal height
  - ❏ the posterior margin of each vertebral body is slightly concave
  - ❏ all three columns appear intact. If any two of the three columns are disrupted then an unstable injury is present
- Lumbar spine. AP projection. Check that the distance between the pedicles widens slightly when descending from L1 to L5.

## THE SUBTLE SIGN NOT TO MISS

| The projection | Finding | Significance |
| --- | --- | --- |
| AP thoracic spine | The soft tissue shadow of the paraspinal line bulges on one (or both) sides | Following trauma this is a localised haematoma – a vertebral fracture is probable |

## REFERENCES

1. Pathria MN, Petersilge CA. Spinal trauma. Radiol Clin North Am 1991; 29: 847–865.
2. Murphey MD, Batritzky S, Bramble JM. Diagnostic imaging of spinal trauma. Radiol Clin North Am 1989; 27: 855–872.
3. Denis F. The three column spine and its significance in the classification of acute thoracolumbar spinal injuries. Spine 1983; 8: 817–831.
4. Genereux GP. The posterior pleural reflections. AJR 1983; 141: 141–149.
5. Donnelly LF, Frush DP, Zheng JY, Biusset GS. Differentiating normal from abnormal inferior thoracic paravertebral soft tissues on chest radiography in children. AJR 2000; 175: 477–483.
6. Berquist TH. Imaging of orthopedic trauma and surgery. Philadelphia, PA: WB Saunders, 1986.
7. Gehweiler JA, Osborne RL, Becker RF. The radiology of vertebral trauma. Philadelphia, PA: WB Saunders, 1980.
8. Daffner RH, Deet ZL, Rothfus WE. The posterior vertebral body line's importance in the detection of burst fractures. AJR 1987; 148: 93–96.

# 10 PELVIS

Pelvic injuries affect two distinct patient groups:

■ A high-velocity injury, typically a road traffic accident.

In this group a minimally displaced fracture can be associated with major organ damage because the forces necessary to cause a fracture of the pelvis are often substantial.[1-4] The sharp edges of cortical bone move inwards and lacerate adjacent organs. The elastic recoil of the tissues may then return the bone fragments to a relatively normal position.[5-7] Plain film radiographs may appear misleadingly reassuring.

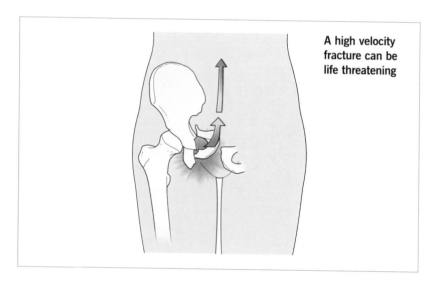

**A high velocity fracture can be life threatening**

■ A low-velocity injury, typically a fall in the street or down the stairs.

In this group a serious soft tissue injury is rare.

## BASIC RADIOGRAPHS

■ AP view only.

This is one of the few sites in the axial or appendicular skeleton where it is standard practice to obtain only one radiograph.

## ANATOMY

■ The pelvis comprises three bone rings (Fig. 10.1):

❑ The main pelvic ring

❑ Two smaller rings formed by the pubic and ischial bones

■ The sturdy sacroiliac joints and the pubic symphysis are part of the main bone ring

■ In children, the synchondrosis (i.e. the cartilaginous junction) between each ischial and pubic bone can sometimes appear confusing (Fig. 10.2). In early childhood these unfused junctions may simulate fracture lines. Subsequently, between the ages of 5 and 7 years the synchondroses may mimic healing fractures.

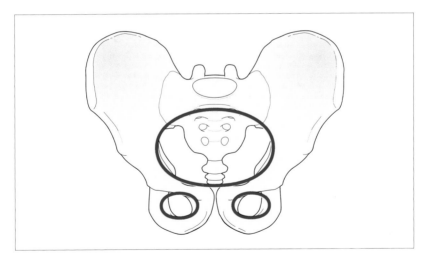

**Figure 10.1** *The pelvis has three rings of bone.*

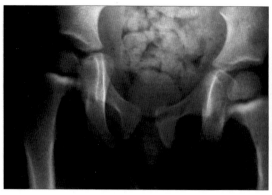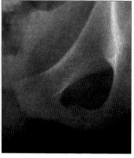

**Figure 10.2** *Normal junction of the ischial and pubic bones in young children. Two different patients. The normal appearance can sometimes be asymmetrical and mimic a fracture or a healing fracture.*

## SYSTEMATIC INSPECTION OF THE AP RADIOGRAPH

*"One fracture in a bone ring is frequently associated with a second fracture"*

Assess:

- The main pelvic ring. Scrutinise both the inner and outer cortices

- The two small rings forming the obturator foramina

- The sacroiliac joints. The widths should be equal (Fig. 10.3)

- The symphysis pubis. The superior surfaces of the body of each pubic bone should align (Fig. 10.3). The maximum width of the joint should be no more than 5 mm

- The sacral foramina (Figs 10.3, 10.4). Disruption of any of the smooth arcuate lines indicates a sacral fracture. Compare the arcs on the injured and uninjured sides

- The region of the acetabulum. This is a complex area and fractures at this site are easy to overlook.[1,7] Compare the injured with the uninjured side.

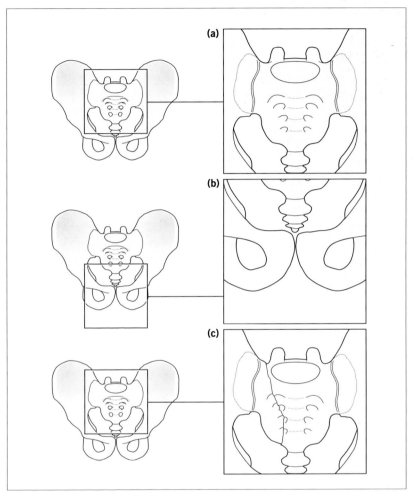

**Figure 10.3** *(a) The width of the sacroiliac joints should be equal. (b) The superior surfaces of the pubic rami should align. (c) The sacral foramina appear as curved (arcuate) white lines. Disruption of the smooth curve of any of these lines indicates a fracture. In this illustration there is a fracture of the right side of the sacrum.*

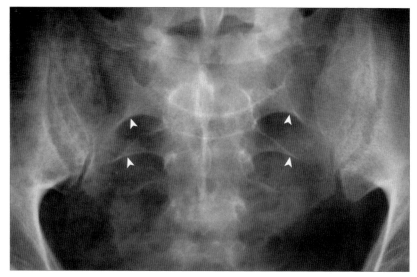

**Figure 10.4** *The normal curved (arcuate) white lines forming the margins of the sacral foramina.*

## FRACTURES
### Involving the main bone ring

■ A fracture through a bone may not be present. Widening (diastasis) at the symphysis pubis (Fig. 10.5) or at a sacroiliac joint constitutes a break in the main pelvic ring (Fig. 10.7)

■ A fracture at one site is likely to be associated with a disruption of the ring at a second site (Fig. 10.6). The second break may be another fracture or it may be ligamentous disruption at the symphysis pubis or at a sacroiliac joint (Fig. 10.5)

■ A double break in the main pelvic ring is an unstable injury.

### Acetabular

Careful scrutiny is essential (Fig. 10.7). They are frequently comminuted.
Bone fragments may be trapped within the joint. These fragments are clinically important. If undetected, and consequently improperly managed, the result may be premature degenerative change.

### Sacral

Often very difficult to detect. The arcuate lines (Figs 10.3, 10.4, 10.8) need to be carefully assessed, comparing one side with the other.

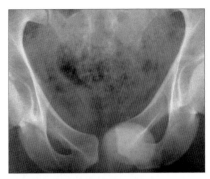

**Figure 10.5** *Disruption of the symphysis pubis. The superior surfaces do not align and the joint is wider than 5 mm.*

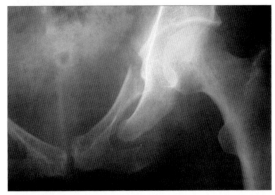

**Figure 10.6** *Although isolated fractures of the small pubic rings do occur it is common for a second fracture to be present.*

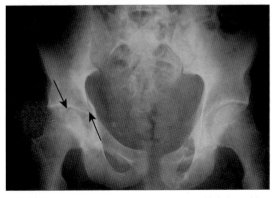

**Figure 10.7** *Fractures of the left superior and inferior pubic rami. A more subtle fracture of the right ischium. These represent fractures of both the main pelvic ring and of the smaller rings. The symphysis pubis is abnormally wide and its margins do not align indicating that there is a second break in the main ring; this pelvis is therefore unstable. Note the acetabular fracture (arrows).*

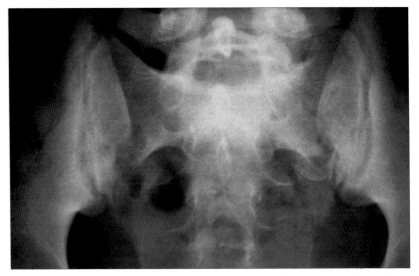

**Figure 10.8** *Fracture through the left side of the sacrum. The foramina are buckled and/or discontinuous. Compare these with the normal smooth curve of the roof of each foramen on the right side.*

## Coccygeal

*History:* Fell on buttocks and the coccyx is tender.

*In practice:* The normal coccyx may appear angulated and very abnormal. In any case, the radiographic findings do not affect management.

*Conclusion:* Radiography is unnecessary.

## Avulsion of an apophysis

These fractures are most commonly caused by repeated or sudden and violent muscle contraction in young people (Figs 10.9, 10.10).

- Sometimes more than one apophysis is avulsed[8–12]

- **Caution**: healing of an avulsion injury may produce considerable ossification/calcification and deformity; either because of wide displacement of the avulsed apophysis or because exuberant healing calcification is laid down. A florid appearance may be mistaken for bone infection or a bone tumour.

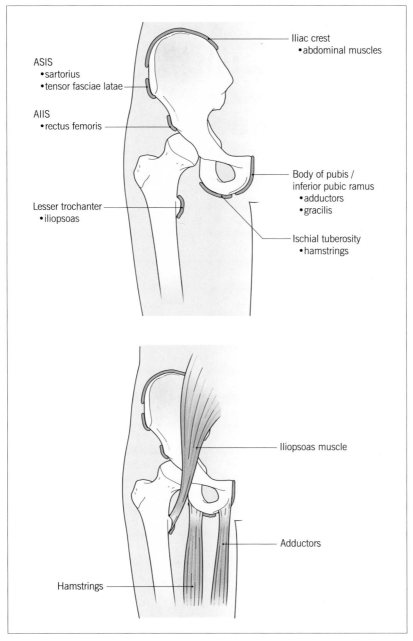

**Figure 10.9** *Normal apophyses – various tendons insert at these sites. In young people a violent muscle contraction can cause an avulsion fracture. AIIS = anterior inferior iliac spine; ASIS = anterior superior iliac spine.*

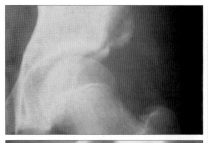

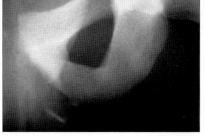

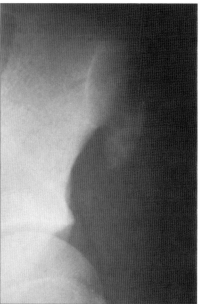

**Figure 10.10** *Avulsed apophyses.*

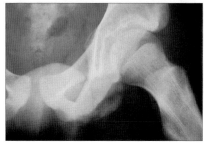

## KEY POINTS

- *Low-velocity injuries in the elderly*: isolated or two fractures of the pubic rami are common. The clinical problem is mainly incapacity due to pain

- *High-velocity injuries*: an apparently minor fracture may be associated with life-threatening soft tissue injury

- Assess the AP radiograph

  - There are three bone rings which frequently fracture at two sites

  - Widening of a sacroiliac joint or of the pubic symphysis may be the site of the second fracture

  - Two fractures in the main ring indicate an unstable injury

- Sacral fractures: the arcuate lines should be smooth – not angulated.

## A SUBTLE SIGN NOT TO MISS – ADULTS

| Presentation | Principle | The search |
|---|---|---|
| Car driver hits oncoming car; complains of pain in knee and pelvis | 'You only see what you look for' | Look through the femoral head for evidence of a subtle fracture of the acetabulum |

## A SUBTLE SIGN NOT TO MISS – ADOLESCENTS

| Presentation | Radiographic appearance | Problem | Diagnosis |
|---|---|---|---|
| Young athlete with pain in region of ischium or symphysis | Rarefaction of bone/moth-eaten appearance/ lucency at site of pain | Misinterpreted as osteomyelitis or Ewing's sarcoma[12] | Chronic avulsion injury due to vigorous muscle contraction:<br>■ Ischium: insertion of the hamstrings<br>■ Symphysis: insertion of the hip adductors |

## REFERENCES

1. Hunter J, Brandser E, Tran K. Pelvic and acetabular trauma. Radiol Clin North Am 1997; 35: 559–590.
2. Rogers LF. Radiology of skeletal trauma, 2nd ed. New York: Churchill Livingstone, 1992; 991–1105.
3. Theumann NH, Verdon JP et al. Traumatic injuries: imaging of pelvic fractures. Eur Radiol 2002; 12: 1312–1320.
4. MacLeod M, Powell J. Evaluation of pelvic fractures: clinical and radiologic. Orthop Clin North Am 1997; 28: 299–319.
5. Young JWR et al. Pelvic fractures: value of plain radiography in the early assessment and management. Radiology 1986; 160: 445–451.
6. Kellam JF, Browner BD. Fractures of the pelvic ring. In: Skeletal trauma. Philadelphia, PA: WB Saunders, 1992; 849–897.
7. Brandser E, Marsh JL. Acetabular fractures: easier classification with a systematic approach. AJR 1998; 171: 1217–1228.
8. Saunders M, Carty H. Avulsion fractures of the pelvis in children: a report of 32 fractures and their outcome. Skeletal Radiol 1994; 23: 85–90.
9. Fernbach SK, Wilkinson RH. Avulsion injuries of the pelvis and proximal femur. AJR 1981; 137: 581–584.
10. Metzmaker JN, Pappas AM. Avulsion fractures of the pelvis. Am J Sports Med 1985; 13: 349–358.
11. El-Khoury GY, Daniel WW, Kathol MH. Acute and chronic avulsive injuries. Radiol Clin North Am 1997; 35: 747–751.
12. Brandser EA, El-Khoury GY, Kathol MH. Adolescent hamstring avulsions that simulate tumours. Emerg Radiol 1995; 2: 273–278.

# 11 HIP AND PROXIMAL FEMUR

Paediatric hip, see page 316.

## BASIC RADIOGRAPHS

- AP of the whole pelvis including both hip joints
- Lateral projection of the painful hip.

## NOTE

- The AP projection allows:

  - Comparison of the injured with the uninjured side

  - Assessment of the pubic rami on the two sides – a pubic ramus fracture can mimic the symptoms and signs of a femoral neck fracture

- A lateral projection of the painful hip is essential. Some femoral neck fractures are impossible to detect on the AP view but may be very obvious on the lateral projection

- Figure 11.1 shows how the femur is positioned for the lateral view, and helps to explain why the subsequent radiographic anatomy (Fig. 11.2) may appear confusing

- Underexposure (film too light) of the lateral radiograph is unacceptable

- Overexposure (film too dark) of the greater trochanter on the AP view is often unavoidable. When this occurs, the area must be examined with a bright light or appropriate windowing (Fig. 11.3).

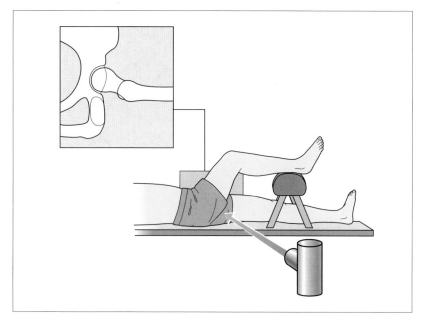

**Figure 11.1** *Technique for the lateral view of the left femoral neck.*

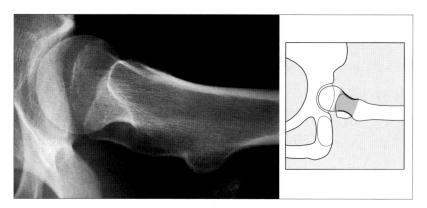

**Figure 11.2** *Lateral view. Normal femoral neck (highlighted in red).*

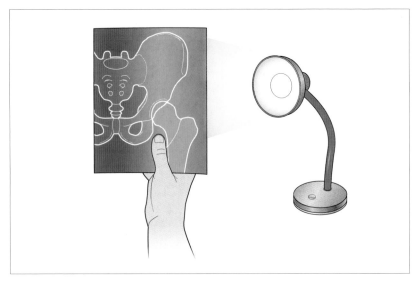

**Figure 11.3** *A bright light (or the correct window level for a digital image) is necessary when assessing the greater trochanter.*

## ANATOMY

■ The femoral neck should have:

❑ A smooth intact cortex – no buckle, no step, no ridge

❑ A normal trabecular pattern (Fig. 11.4)

❑ No transverse areas of sclerosis

■ The intertrochanteric region should have:

❑ An appearance identical to the same area on the opposite femur

❑ No black or lucent line crossing the intertrochanteric bone nor interrupting the cortical margin of the greater trochanter.

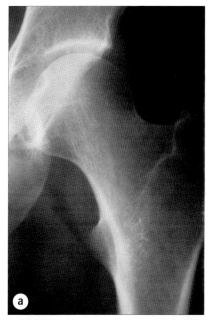

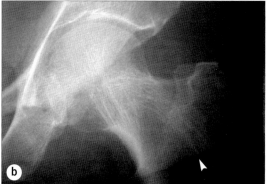

**Figure 11.4** *AP view. Normal hips. Two different patients (a) and (b). The cortical margins are smooth and there are no sclerotic (dense) transverse lines. The normal weight-bearing trabeculae are prominent in (b); less prominent in (a). The visibility of the trabecular pattern varies between patients. Note the skin fold crossing the femur (b). A skin fold can sometimes mimic a fracture, but a fold will continue outwards across the radiograph and away from the bone.*

## INJURIES

### FRACTURES

#### Proximal femur

- Fractures of the femoral neck and proximal femur[1,2] occur at characteristic sites (Figs 11.5–11.7)

- Most fractures are widely displaced and easy to detect

- A few fractures are very difficult to detect (Fig. 11.8). If the radiographs appear superficially normal it is important to answer the following questions:

  - Are the cortical margins of the femoral neck continuous or is there a slight step?

  - Is the trabecular pattern continuous, or is it interrupted?

  - Does a dense white line (compression or impaction of bone) cross the femoral neck?

- Occasionally, an undisplaced fracture will be undetectable on the initial radiographs. If there is strong clinical suspicion of a fracture then referral for MRI or radionuclide study is indicated.

---

**Pitfall 1:** An acetabular fracture may be accompanied by similar clinical features to a fracture of the femoral neck. These fractures are very easy to overlook.[3,4] Careful scrutiny is essential (see Fig. 10.7).

---

**Pitfall 2:** A fracture of a pubic ramus (Fig. 11.9) can present with symptoms identical to a fracture of the femoral neck. In practice, the commonest pelvic fracture following a fall in an elderly patient is an isolated fracture of the superior pubic ramus.

---

**Pitfall 3:** In the elderly, a ring of osteophytes (Fig. 11.10) around the acetabular margin can produce a dense white line across the femoral neck; this may mimic an impacted fracture.

---

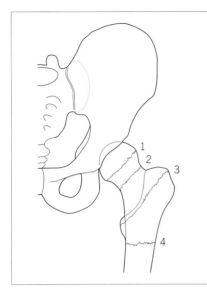

**Figure 11.5** *Fractures of the proximal femur. The site of fracture affects both prognosis and management.[1,2] Characteristic sites: subcapital 1, transcervical 2, intertrochanteric 3, subtrochanteric 4. Fractures 1 and 2 are intracapsular; fractures 3 and 4 are extracapsular. An extracapsular fracture does not run the risk of avascular necrosis and, consequently, internal fixation invariably produces a good outcome.*

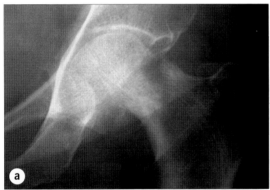

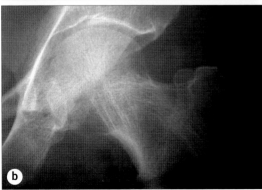

**Figure 11.6** *The subcapital fracture **(a)** is identified by the break in the cortical outline and the interruption in the white lines that represent the weight-bearing trabeculae. Compare this appearance with uninterrupted and normal trabeculae **(b)**.*

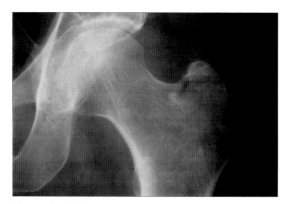

**Figure 11.7** *Fracture of the greater trochanter.*

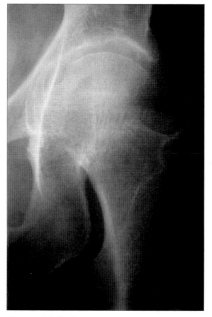

**Figure 11.8** *The sclerotic (dense) line indicates an impacted subcapital fracture.*

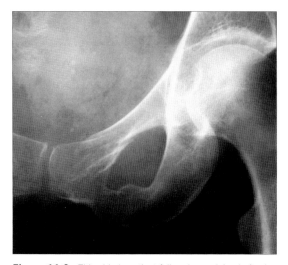

**Figure 11.9** *This elderly patient fell and complained of pain in the hip. A femoral neck fracture was suspected. The femoral neck is intact but there are fractures of the superior and inferior pubic rami. This clinical history and these radiological findings are a common occurrence.*

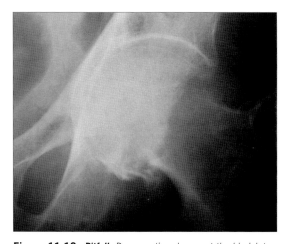

**Figure 11.10** *Pitfall: Degenerative change at the hip joint. A ring of osteophytes around the margin of the acetabulum produces sclerosis across the femoral neck. Sometimes this appearance can mimic a subcapital fracture.*

## DISLOCATIONS

■ Dislocations can be posterior, anterior, or central; 80% are posterior (Fig. 11.11)

■ These injuries result from high impact trauma

   ❑ The AP view usually demonstrates the dislocation

   ❑ Fractures of the acetabular margin are a common complication of posterior dislocation. An unrecognised fragment may prevent reduction – or cause instability if the acetabular defect is large.

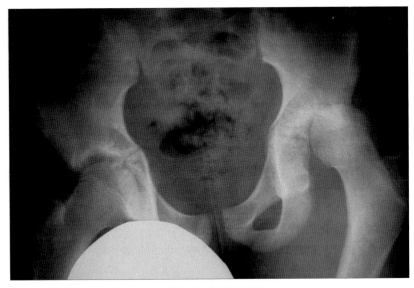

**Figure 11.11** *Posterior dislocation of the head of the left femur.*

## KEY POINTS

- An AP view of the whole pelvis is mandatory
  - ❏ It allows comparison with the uninjured side
  - ❏ A fracture through a pubic ramus may mimic the pain of a femoral neck fracture
- A lateral view is essential. A fracture involving the femoral neck and/or the trochanteric region may be detectable on this projection only
- A dense white line may be the only evidence of an impacted fracture of the femoral neck
- Some areas on the radiographs will often be slightly overexposed. These must be scrutinised with a bright light or careful windowing.

## THE SUBTLE SIGN NOT TO MISS

| History | AP radiograph | Significance |
|---------|---------------|--------------|
| Road traffic accident – front seat passenger has sustained a dashboard injury | Linear density projected over the femoral head | The density is a fragment detached from the acetabulum.[3] An important injury |

## REFERENCES

1. Parker MJ, Pryor GA. Hip fracture management. Oxford: Blackwell Scientific, 1993.
2. Otremski I, Katz A, Dekel S *et al*. Natural history of impacted subcapital femoral fractures and its relevance to treatment options. Injury 1990; 21: 379–381.
3. Rogers LF *et al*. Occult central fractures of the acetabulum. AJR 1975; 124: 96–101.
4. Brandser E, Marsh JL. Acetabular fractures: easier classification with a systematic approach. AJR 1998; 171: 1217–1228.

# 12 KNEE

The majority of knee injuries affect the soft tissues (i.e. cartilages and ligaments). In most instances the bones will be normal.

Extensively tested guidelines have resulted in the Ottawa knee rules for requesting radiography.[1]

## BASIC RADIOGRAPHS

### ALL INJURIES

- AP

- Lateral – obtained with the patient supine and using a horizontal X-ray beam (Fig. 12.1)

- Other additional projections are occasionally useful.[2,3]

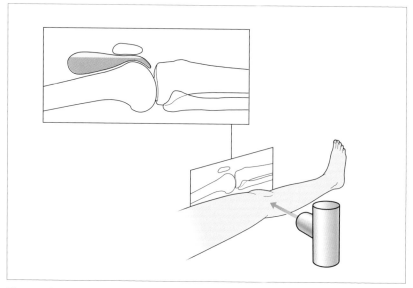

**Figure 12.1** *In the Emergency Department the lateral view of the knee is obtained with a horizontal X-ray beam. In this patient a fat–fluid level is present. Fat (light shading) lies on top of blood (dark shading) in the suprapatellar bursa.*

## PATELLAR INJURY

■ If the AP and lateral radiographs appear normal and there is continuing clinical suspicion of a patellar fracture then oblique or skyline views are indicated

■ If an osteochondral fracture of the articular surface of the patella is suspected (e.g. following a patellar dislocation) then a skyline view is necessary.

## ANATOMY

■ The tibial plateau. A useful rule:

*On the AP view a perpendicular line drawn at the most lateral margin of the femoral condyle should not have more than 5 mm of the lateral margin of the tibial condyle outside of it* (Fig. 12.2)

This measurement is relevant to fractures of the lateral tibial plateau. A similar rule can be applied to the relationship between the medial femoral condyle and the medial tibial plateau

■ The patella may develop from several ossification centres. Sometimes these centres remain unfused in the adult. The most common variant is two centres (bipartite patella). The smaller unfused centre will have a corticated margin and is characteristically positioned in the upper outer quadrant (Fig. 12.3). Occasionally there are three unfused ossification centres (i.e. a tripartite patella)

■ The normal position of the patella. A useful rule:

*On the lateral radiograph the distance from the tibial tubercle (on the anterior aspect of the tibia) to the lower pole of the patella should approximate to the length of the patella itself ±20%* (Fig. 12.4)

This rule has a relevance to rupture of the patellar ligament[3–5]

■ The fabella is a common sesamoid bone in the tendon of the lateral head of the gastrocnemius muscle. Its posterior position is characteristic (Fig. 12.5). It should not be confused with a fracture fragment or a loose body.

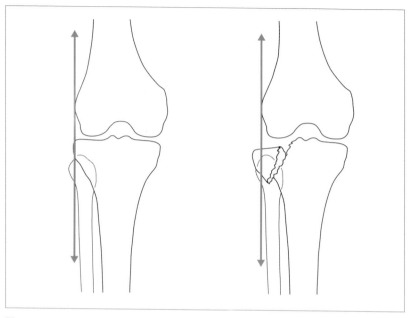

**Figure 12.2** *In the normal knee (left) a perpendicular line drawn at the most lateral margin of the femur should have no more than 5 mm of adjacent tibia outside of it. Following trauma, if this rule is broken a plateau fracture should be suspected.*

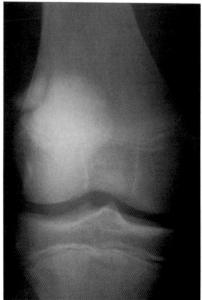

**Figure 12.3** *Bipartite patella in an adolescent. This is a normal variant and should not be confused with a fracture. The margins are sclerotic and well defined. The position in the upper outer quadrant is characteristic. This common variant can be seen in old and young people.*

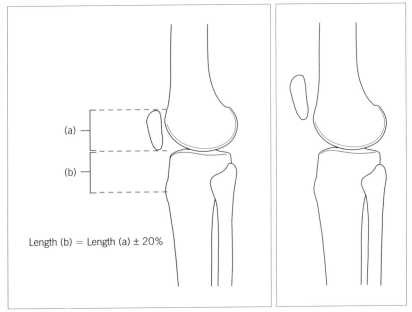

**Figure 12.4** *Patellar rule: 'the distance from the tibial tubercle (on the anterior aspect of the tibia) to the lower pole of the patella should approximate to the length of the patella – plus or minus 20%'. When this rule is broken, a rupture of the patellar ligament must be excluded. Normal on the left. Ruptured ligament on the right.*

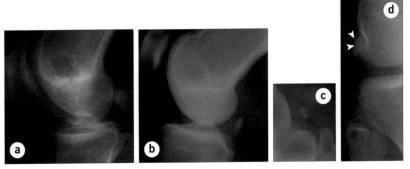

**Figure 12.5** *The fabella is a sesamoid bone in the tendon of the lateral head of the gastrocnemius muscle. Sometimes its shape and position is not altogether characteristic. Examples: **(a)** is characteristic; **(b)** a somewhat craggy looking fabella; **(c)** a bipartite or double fabella; **(d)** the normal fabella may be situated in a seemingly far lateral position.*

## INJURIES

### SOFT TISSUE

- Most patients who sustain a severe ligamentous or meniscal injury have normal radiographs

- A large effusion will be apparent on the lateral radiograph as an oval soft tissue density posterior to the quadriceps tendon

- Rupture of the patellar tendon is identified by a high position of the patella on the lateral radiograph (Fig. 12.6). The rule: *in the normal patient the distance from the tibial tubercle to the lower pole of the patella should not exceed the length of the patella by more than 20%.*

---

**Pitfall:** Soft tissue calcification adjacent to the medial epicondyle of the femur should not be mistaken for a fracture fragment. The calcification is termed a Pellegrini–Stieda lesion (Fig. 12.7). It represents calcification following a previous old sprain of the medial collateral ligament.

---

### FRACTURES

**General**

- Most fractures are easy to detect

- Lipohaemarthrosis. Occasionally, the only sign of an intra-articular fracture will be a fat–fluid level on the lateral radiograph. This appearance is only seen on a lateral view obtained with a horizontal beam (Figs 12.1, 12.8)

  - An effusion in the suprapatellar bursa may contain fat released from the bone marrow. The fat layers on top of the underlying fluid (blood) resulting in a fat–fluid level

  - A fat–fluid level (FFL) is sometimes referred to as a fat–blood interface, or FBI. It indicates an intra-articular fracture. Even if a fracture is not identified, assume that an undisplaced fracture is present.

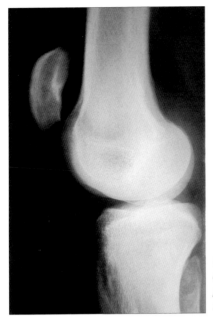

**Figure 12.6** *High position of the patella. Rupture of the patellar ligament. The patellar rule (Figure 12.4) is broken.*

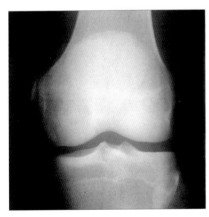

**Figure 12.7** *A previous sprain of the medial collateral ligament has resulted in Pellegrini–Stieda calcification. Not a fracture. The position of the calcification adjacent to the medial femoral condyle is characteristic.*

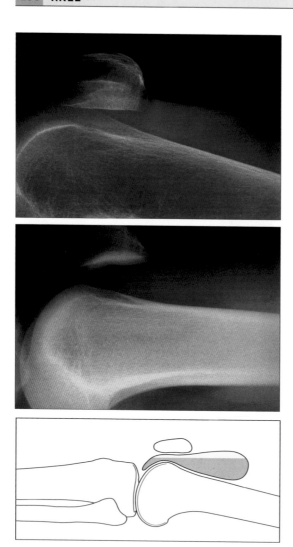

**Figure 12.8** *Fat–fluid level in the suprapatellar bursa. A fat–fluid level indicates an intra-articular fracture – even if a fracture is not identified.*

## Accompanying a cruciate ligament injury

The cruciate ligaments insert into the intercondylar region (i.e. anteriorly and posteriorly) of the tibial plateau. When a rupture occurs it is occasionally complicated by a fracture.

■ If a fracture of the intercondylar eminence (i.e. the tibial spine) is identified then this is commonly consequent on an avulsion of the tibial attachment of the anterior cruciate ligament. Occasionally, the detached bone fragment may be loose and visible within the joint (Fig. 12.9). An avulsed bone fragment is most often seen in adolescents; it is exceptionally rare in adults

■ The lateral capsular sign (or Segond fracture) is a small avulsion fracture of the margin of the lateral tibial plateau just below the joint line (Fig. 12.10). This fracture has a strong association with a tear of the anterior cruciate ligament and meniscal injuries.[6,7]

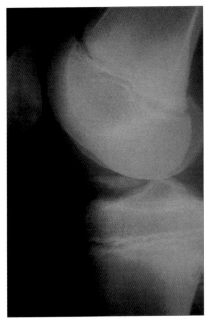

**Figure 12.9** *Avulsion fracture at the insertion of the anterior cruciate ligament. The large fragment lies anteriorly within the joint.*

## Involving a tibial plateau

These fractures (Figs 12.11, 12.12) are often associated with significant damage to the medial collateral ligament or cruciate ligaments.

■ 80% involve the lateral plateau. They are usually seen as a depression in the plateau following violent impaction from the lateral femoral condyle. This is the so-called 'car bumper' or 'fender' fracture (Fig. 12.13). A similar injury to the medial plateau is less frequent (Fig. 12.14). The latter results from forced impaction from the medial femoral condyle

■ **Useful clue 1:** Evidence of an impacted fracture may be subtle. It may show an area of increased density due to bone compression (Figs 12.11, 12.13, 12.15). Oblique views may be very useful in confirming the diagnosis

■ **Useful clue 2:** The tibial margin is often displaced as a result of a fracture of the lateral plateau (Fig. 12.15). The rule to be applied:

*'a perpendicular line drawn at the most lateral margin of the femur should not have more than 5 mm of the adjacent margin of the tibia beyond it'* (Fig. 12.2)

If this rule is broken a plateau fracture should be suspected.

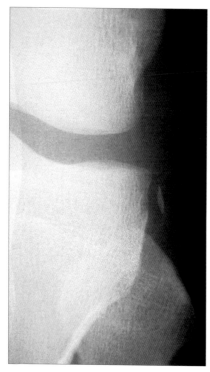

**Figure 12.10** *Small fracture – important connotations. This Segond fracture is an avulsion fracture. The fragment has a characteristic position adjacent to the lateral tibial plateau just below the joint line. There is a strong association with an injury to the anterior cruciate ligament or to a meniscus.*

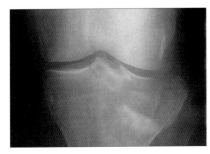

**Figure 12.11** *Fracture of the lateral tibial plateau. A full house of radiographic signs: the fracture line, the dense (sclerotic) area indicating impaction, the lateral displacement of the margin of the tibia.*

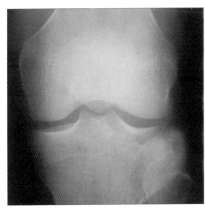

**Figure 12.12** *Fracture of the lateral tibial plateau. The area of sclerosis (density) is due to bone impaction.*

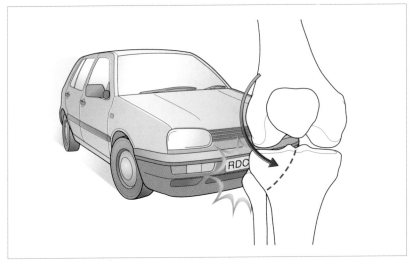

**Figure 12.13** *A blow to the outside of the knee joint is the cause of a fracture of the lateral tibial plateau.*

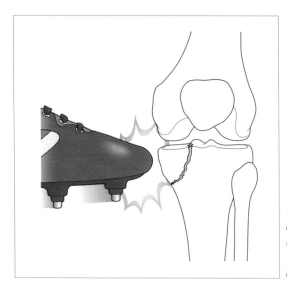

**Figure 12.14** *A fracture of the medial tibial plateau is much less common than a 'fender' fracture of the lateral plateau.*

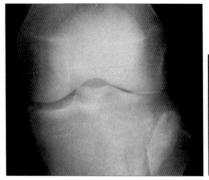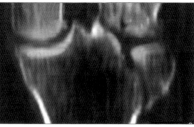

**Figure 12.15** *Tibial plateau fracture. The plain radiographs invariably show that a fracture has occurred. Nevertheless, the findings may be subtle. In this patient there is a faint fracture line, an area of sclerosis due to impaction, and lateral displacement of the margin of the tibia (the 5 mm rule is broken). Most patients will require a CT or MRI examination in order to show the surgeon the extent of the bone injury and the amount of displacement and depression of the articular surface.*

## Patella

*General*

■ A direct blow is the usual cause of a fracture. Vertical, horizontal and comminuted fractures occur (Figs 12.16, 12.17)

■ Violent contraction of the quadriceps muscle can cause a transverse fracture in an athlete

■ Occasionally, a fracture will not be shown on either of the standard views. This is usually a vertical fracture. Clinical suspicion and concern will determine whether a further view – either an oblique[2,8] or skyline view (Fig. 12.18) – is necessary

■ An unfused secondary ossification centre – a bipartite patella – in the upper outer quadrant may mimic a fracture (Fig. 12.3). An ossification centre will have a well defined sclerotic (corticated) edge and its margin will match the contour of the adjacent bone.

*Osteochondral fracture of an articular surface*

■ This is a recognised complication of patellar dislocation and results from shearing or impaction

■ It involves the medial surface of the patella or the lateral femoral condyle (Fig. 12.19)

■ Sometimes the defect in the articular surface is only shown on a skyline view.[3,8]

## Neck of fibula

These fractures (Fig. 12.20) should not be dismissed lightly. Isolated fractures of the head or neck of the fibula do occur. Nevertheless, they are often associated with a severe knee injury including damage to the collateral or cruciate ligaments.[6,9]

## Tibial tubercle

■ Avulsion of the tubercle in a child is not a diagnosis easily made on plain films alone. The normal appearance may be alarming (Fig. 12.21). In general, assessment is best made on the clinical findings, particularly in children with chronic pain

■ Osgood–Schlatter's disease results from recurrent episodes of minor trauma,[11,12] most commonly in adolescent boys. A plain film diagnosis cannot be made with absolute certainty because the normal ossification centre can appear very fragmented, irregular, or separate (Fig. 12.21). This diagnosis is best made on clinical history and examination.

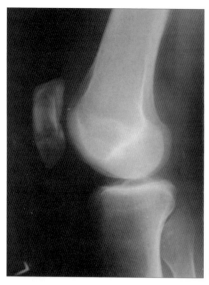

**Figure 12.16** *Comminuted fracture of the patella.*

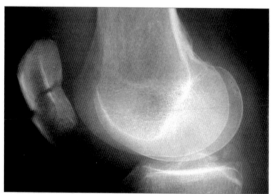

**Figure 12.17** *Transverse fracture of the patella.*

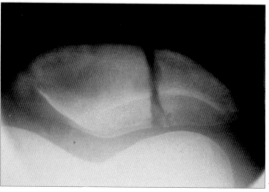

**Figure 12.18** *A few patellar fractures are impossible to identify on the standard AP and lateral views. If there is clinical suspicion of a patellar injury and standard radiographs appear normal then an additional view of the patella should be obtained – a skyline or an oblique projection.*

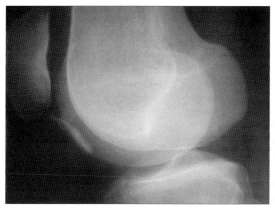

**Figure 12.19** *Osteochondral fracture due to a shearing/impaction injury. An unusually large fragment lies in the joint. This radiograph does not indicate from which articular surface it has originated.*

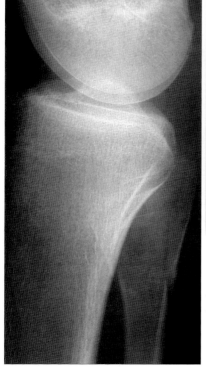

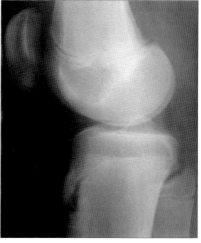

**Figure 12.21** *Normal tibial tubercle. Sometimes the fragmentation or irregularity at this site is gross and yet still within the normal range. Osgood–Schlatter's disease cannot be reliably diagnosed or excluded by radiography. The diagnosis is made on clinical findings.*

**Figure 12.20** *Another small fracture that may have an important connotation. An isolated fracture of the neck of the fibula may be associated with damage to the collateral or cruciate ligaments.*

## KEY POINTS

- Most fractures are obvious

- A normal radiograph does not exclude severe ligamentous or cartilaginous injury

- A fat–fluid level (FFL or FBI) in the suprapatellar bursa on the lateral film indicates an intra-articular fracture

- Tibial plateau fractures can be very subtle. Look for:
  - An area of increased bone density
  - Displacement of the margin of the tibia

- Patellar fractures. If the AP and lateral films appear normal and there is continuing clinical concern, oblique or skyline views are indicated.

## SUBTLE SIGNS NOT TO MISS

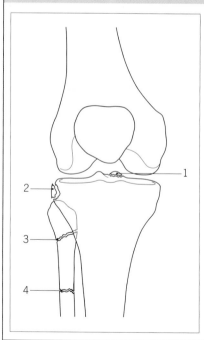

A small fracture around the knee joint may indicate an important injury elsewhere:

1. *Intercondylar eminence*
   Cruciate ligament injury

2. *Segond fracture*
   Tear of the anterior cruciate ligament and/or meniscal injury

3. *Neck of fibula*
   Injury to the collateral or cruciate ligaments

4. *Proximal third of shaft of fibula*
   Maisonneuve fracture – an associated ankle fracture

## REFERENCES

1. Stiell IG, Wells GA, Hoag RH *et al*. Implementation of the Ottawa knee rule for the use of radiography in acute knee injuries. JAMA 1997; 278: 2075–2079.
2. Daffner RH, Tabas JH. Trauma oblique radiographs of the knee. J Bone Joint Surg 1987; 69A: 568–571.
3. Capps GW, Hayes CW. Easily missed injuries around the knee. Radiographics 1994; 14: 1191–1210.
4. Insall J, Salvati E. Patella position in the normal knee joint. Radiology 1971; 101: 101–104.
5. Newberg A, Wales L. Radiographic diagnosis of quadriceps tendon rupture. Radiology 1977; 125: 367–371.
6. Goldman AB, Pavlow H, Rubenstein D. The Segond fracture of the proximal tibia. A small avulsion that reflects major ligamentous damage. AJR 1988; 151: 1163–1167.
7. Dietz GW, Wilcox DM, Montgomery JB. Segond tibial condyle fracture: lateral capsular ligament avulsion. Radiology 1986; 159: 467–469.
8. Rorabeck CH, Bobbechko WP. Acute dislocation of the patella with osteochondral fracture: a review of eighteen cases. J Bone Joint Surg 1976; 58B: 237–240.
9. El-Khoury GY, Daniel WW, Kathol MH. Acute and chronic avulsive injuries. Radiol Clin North Am 1997; 35: 747–766.
10. Ogden JA, Tross RB, Murphy MJ. Fractures of the tibial tuberosity in adolescents. J Bone Joint Surg 1980; 62A: 205–215.
11. Rosenberg ZS, Kawelblum M, Cheung YY *et al*. Osgood–Schlatter's lesion: fracture or tendinitis? Scintigraphic, CT, and MR imaging features. Radiology 1992; 185: 853–858.
12. Kujala UM, Kvist M, Heinonen O. Osgood–Schlatter's disease in adolescent athletes. Retrospective study of incidence and duration. Am J Sports Med 1985; 13: 236–241.

# 13 ANKLE AND HINDFOOT

The ankle is a ring structure of three bones (tibia, talus and fibula) linked by three ligaments (the medial and lateral collateral ligaments and the interosseous ligament). A break in one part of the ring is likely to result in a second break elsewhere. The second break may be another fracture or a ligamentous injury – either a sprain, a tear, or a rupture.

The hindfoot comprises the talus and the calcaneum and their articulations with the navicular and cuboid bones.

Requests for ankle radiography are particularly common in the ED. Numerous decision rules have been suggested. Application of the Ottawa ankle rules[1,2] has been shown to produce a significant reduction in unnecessary ankle radiography.

## BASIC RADIOGRAPHS

### ANKLE INJURY

- **AP mortice:** obtained with slight (20°) internal rotation so that the fibula does not overlap the talus (Fig. 13.1)
- **Lateral:** to include the entire calcaneum and its anterior process. Ideally, the base of the fifth metatarsal will be included (Fig. 13.2).

### CALCANEAL INJURY

- **Lateral:** to include the ankle and hindfoot (Fig. 13.2)
- **Axial:** aka the tangential projection (Figs 13.3, 13.4).

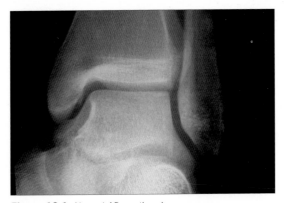

**Figure 13.1** *Normal AP mortice view.*

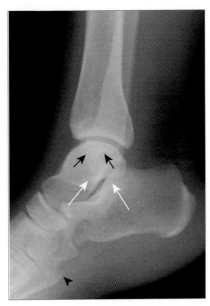

**Figure 13.2** *Normal lateral view. The lateral malleolus (white arrows) is projected inferior to the medial malleolus (black arrows). Note that the entire calcaneum and the base of the fifth metatarsal (arrowhead) are included on the radiograph.*

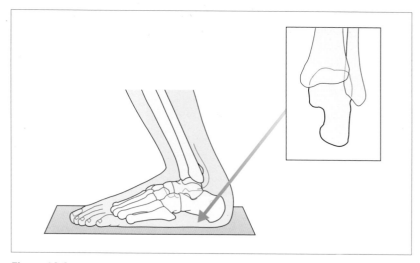

**Figure 13.3** *Technique for obtaining the axial view of the calcaneum. This radiographic projection can be obtained with the patient lying down (or standing).*

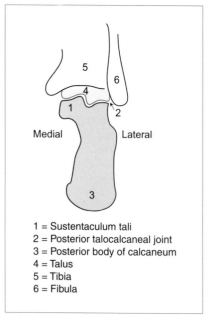

1 = Sustentaculum tali
2 = Posterior talocalcaneal joint
3 = Posterior body of calcaneum
4 = Talus
5 = Tibia
6 = Fibula

**Figure 13.4** *The anatomical structures visualised on the axial view of the calcaneum. In practice, the anterior aspect of the calcaneum is never as clearly demonstrated as the posterior aspect.*

## ANATOMY

### AP MORTICE PROJECTION

- The joint space should be of uniform width all the way around (Fig. 13.1).
  It can be traced along its medial side, over the superior aspect (i.e. the dome)
  of the talus, on to the lateral side of the joint

- The surface of the talar dome should be smooth. No irregularity

- The width (Fig. 13.5) of the space between the distal tibia and fibula. When
  measured at a point 1.0 cm proximal to the tibial plafond (i.e. the articular
  surface) this space should not be more than 6 mm wide.[3]

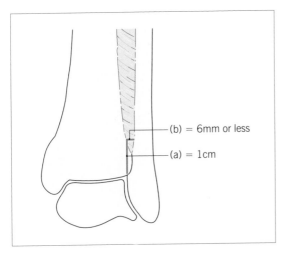

(b) = 6mm or less

(a) = 1cm

**Figure 13.5** *Assessing
the interosseous ligament
(between the tibia and fibula).
A useful rule of thumb: at a
point 1.0 cm proximal to the
articular surface of the tibia
the space between tibia and
fibula should not exceed 6 mm.
If this is exceeded – suspect a
tear or rupture of the ligament.*

### LATERAL PROJECTION

- The lateral and medial malleoli can be identified (Fig. 13.2). The lateral malleolus
  extends more inferiorly than the medial malleolus. The medial malleolus has a
  notch; this assists with identification

- The posterior aspect of the tibia, conventionally (but inaccurately) referred to as
  the posterior malleolus, is well shown

- The calcaneum and its sustentaculum tali are demonstrated (Fig. 13.2)

- The base of the fifth metatarsal is often included.

## AXIAL PROJECTION: THE CALCANEUM

■ The posterior two thirds of the bone is well shown

■ The sustentaculum tali is often slightly under-exposed (Figs 13.4, 13.6).

## NOTE: THE ACCESSORY OSSICLES

■ Small bones (Fig. 13.7) lying adjacent to the tips of the medial and lateral malleoli are very common. They may be misdiagnosed as avulsed fracture fragments. Sometimes difficult to distinguish from a fracture and clinical correlation is important. Fractures are tender, accessory ossicles are not. Also:

❑ An accessory ossicle has a well defined (i.e. corticated) outline

❑ An acute fracture fragment is ill defined (i.e. not corticated) on one of its sides

■ Os trigonum. A small bone closely applied to the posterior aspect of the talus is common. It can be separate from the talus or fused to it; it may be small or large (Fig. 13.8); it is sometimes multiple. Occasionally it is misread as a fracture fragment.

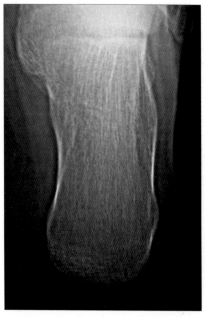

**Figure 13.6** *Axial view of the calcaneum. Normal. The anatomical aspects are explained in Fig. 13.4.*

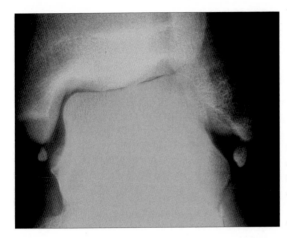

**Figure 13.7** *The small bones adjacent to the tip of the lateral and medial malleoli have well corticated margins. These are unfused secondary centres.*

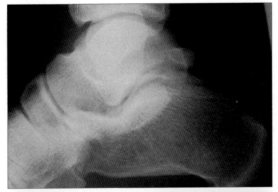

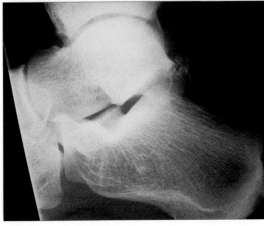

**Figure 13.8** *Normal (varying) appearances of the os trigonum. See text.*

## FRACTURES

### Epiphyseal plate (Salter–Harris) fractures

Common injuries in children. The distal tibia and fibula are frequently affected. Growth plate fractures are described on pages 306–309.

### The malleoli

These fractures are usually obvious. However:

- A fracture may be identified on one view only (Figs 13.9, 13.10). For this reason the lateral projection must be scrutinised particularly carefully – especially for oblique fractures of the fibula, and for fractures involving the posterior aspect of the tibia (Fig. 13.10)

- If one fracture is seen then it is necessary to look for a second fracture or joint space widening (ligamentous damage).

---

## Ankle slip-ups

1. If both projections are not scrutinised carefully it is possible for an important but undisplaced fracture of the tibia to be misdiagnosed as a less serious fibula fracture (Fig. 13.11).

2. Maisonneuve fracture. The ankle joint is in effect a bone ring. The ring extends as high as the knee. An external rotation injury of the ankle may result in a high fracture of the proximal shaft of the fibula. The fibular fracture may be overlooked because the main symptoms are around the ankle joint (Fig. 13.12). This combination of injuries is known as a Maisonneuve fracture.

   - Suspect this injury when the radiographs show an isolated fracture of the medial malleolus accompanied by widening of the medial joint space; or when clinical examination of the upper leg is painful

   - Examine the upper leg in all patients attending with an ankle injury.

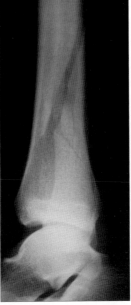

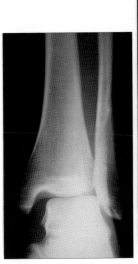

**Figure 13.9** *The AP mortice view shows widening of the medial joint space indicating damage to the medial collateral ligament. Since the bone–ligamentous ring has been ruptured at one position then a second injury should be sought. The lateral view shows an oblique fracture of the fibula.*

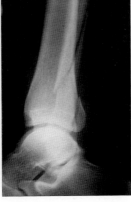

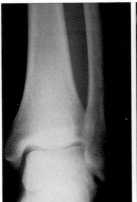

**Figure 13.10** *This AP mortice view could be considered to be normal. The lateral projection reveals obvious oblique fractures of the fibula and of the posterior aspect of the tibia. The rule: "evaluating one view only is one view too few".*

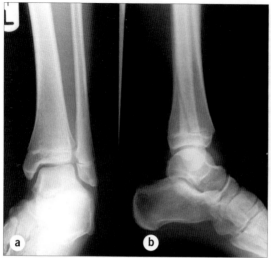

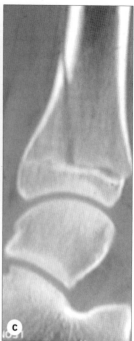

**Figure 13.11** *(a) AP view shows no abnormality. (b) lateral view. A fracture is clearly visable. This was incorrectly interpreted as a fibular fracture. (c) CT-reformatted image shows oblique fracture of the tibia with widening of the epiphysis anteriorly (Salter – Harris type 2 fracture)*

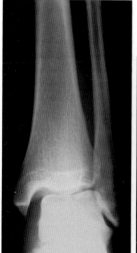

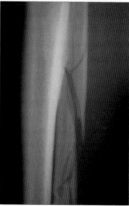

**Figure 13.12** *Maisonneuve fracture. Widening of the medial aspect of the ankle joint. No other bone or ligamentous injury shown around the ankle joint. The ankle joint is in effect a bone ring. In this instance, the second injury is a fracture of the midshaft of the fibula.*

## The talus

*Osteochondral fractures*

Small but clinically important impaction fractures. They usually occur during inversion.[4,5]

- Often involve the medial or lateral aspect of the talar dome
- Identified as a defect or an irregularity of the cortex (Fig. 13.13)
- Sometimes the small fragment becomes detached and lies free within the joint.

*Neck of the talus[6]*

- An important injury because of the high risk of subsequent avascular necrosis and secondary degenerative arthritis
- A displaced fracture is easy to detect. An undisplaced fracture is easy to overlook (Fig. 13.14).

*Body of the talus[6]*

- Delay in diagnosis/treatment can lead to painful non-union or subtalar-osteoarthritis
- Fractures can occur in the coronal, sagittal or horizontal planes
- A fracture through the lateral process of the talus is frequently overlooked. Scrutinising this area on the AP view is essential following all inversion injuries (Fig. 13.15).

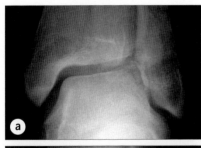

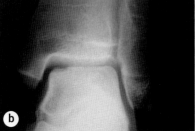

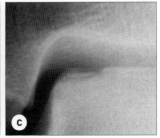

**Figure 13.13** *Osteochondral fractures of the talar dome. Two different patients. The lateral aspect of the dome is disrupted (a). Fracture of the medial aspect (b,c).*

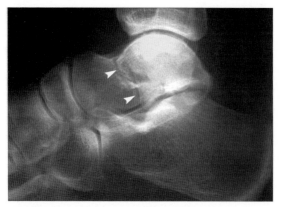

**Figure 13.14** *Fracture through the neck of the talus.*

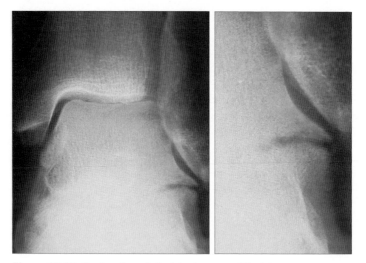

**Figure 13.15** *Fracture through the lateral process of the talus.*

## The calcaneum

- The calcaneum is the most commonly injured bone of the hindfoot

- Most severe injuries occur following a fall from a height (Fig. 13.16). If a calcaneal fracture is suspected clinically then an axial view should be obtained (Fig. 13.17)

- Some fractures, particularly those involving the anterior process of the calcaneum, can result from an apparently simple twisting injury.

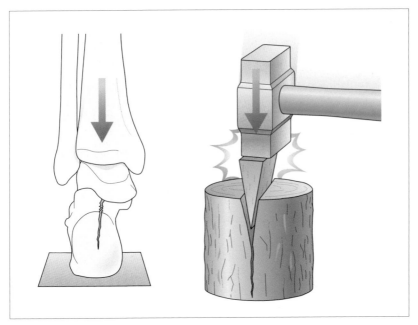

**Figure 13.16** *Fall from a height. Fracture through the body of the calcaneum. The fracture partly results from the talus driving into the calcaneum. This effect can be likened to a wedge slamming into a block of wood.*

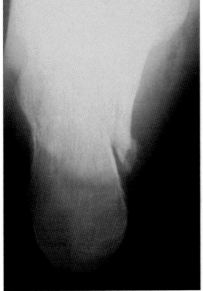

**Figure 13.17** *Axial view of the calcaneum showing a fracture.*

*Types of calcaneal fracture[5,6]*

- **Intra-articular** (75%)
  - ❑ Involve the subtalar or calcaneocuboid joints
  - ❑ Some fractures will only become apparent when Bohler's angle is assessed on the lateral view (Fig. 13.18). This angle is normally 30–40°. If the fracture results in flattening of the bone then the angle will be less than 30° (Figs 13.19 and 13.20)
  - ❑ A sclerotic line or density in the body of the calcaneum may be the only evidence of an impacted fracture (Fig. 13.21)

- **Extra-articular** (25%)
  - ❑ Usually more difficult to detect compared with intra-articular fractures
  - ❑ An anterior process fracture[6,7] is the most common (Fig. 13.22). Usually well shown on the lateral radiograph
  - ❑ Fatigue fractures occur. They result from repetitive stress/trauma. Usually identified as an area of bone sclerosis.

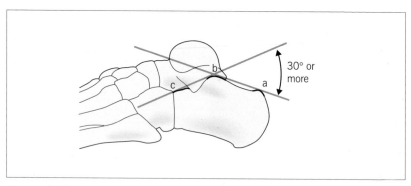

**Figure 13.18** *Normal Bohler's angle. This is assessed on the lateral radiograph. It is measured by drawing a line from the posterior aspect of the calcaneum to its highest midpoint (line ab). A second line is then drawn from point (b) to the highest anterior point (c). The angle to be measured is shown.*

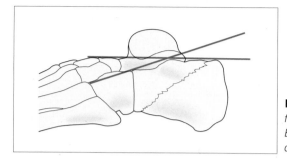

**Figure 13.19** *Calcaneal fracture with compression. Bohler's angle (normally 30° or more) is flattened.*

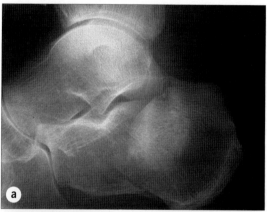

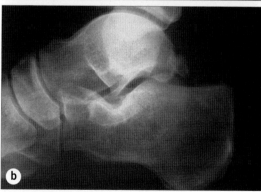

**Figure 13.20** *Calcaneal fractures. (a) A linear fracture, impaction sclerosis, and Bohler's angle is flattened. (b) The only evidence of a calcaneal fracture is the flattened Bohler's angle.*

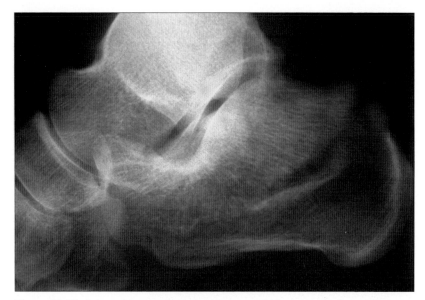

**Figure 13.21** *Calcaneal fracture. Bohler's angle is normal. The fracture is shown mainly as areas of impaction sclerosis adjacent to a linear fracture line.*

**Figure 13.22** *Fracture of the anterior process of the calcaneum. This particular fracture usually results from a twisting injury and not from a fall from a height. As a consequence, this fracture will sometimes be detected on an oblique radiograph of the foot – obtained because of a suspected midfoot injury.*

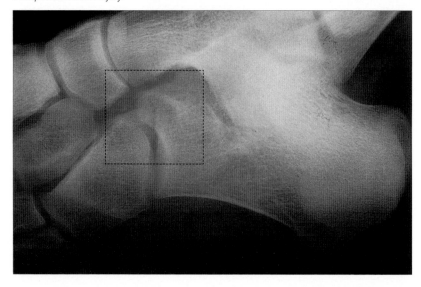

## Base of the fifth metatarsal

*Avulsion fracture of the tuberosity*

■ This common injury results from avulsion of the metatarsal tuberosity at the insertion of the peroneus brevis tendon (Fig. 13.23). The fracture (Fig. 13.24) occurs as a consequence of forced inversion

■ An inversion injury does not warrant a routine request for ankle and foot radiography. Careful clinical examination of the base of the fifth metatarsal will indicate when radiographs of the foot should be obtained.

---

### Pitfalls

1. In young patients the normal unfused apophysis (Fig. 13.25) at the base of the fifth metatarsal should not be misinterpreted as a fracture. Apply this rule:

   "a fracture fragment usually lies transverse to the long axis of the metatarsal whereas an apophysis lies in the long axis of the metatarsal" (Fig. 13.26).

2. Jones' fracture[6]. Often confused with an avulsion injury. It must be treated differently to an avulsion of the tuberosity. See: Midfoot and Forefoot, Chapter 14.

---

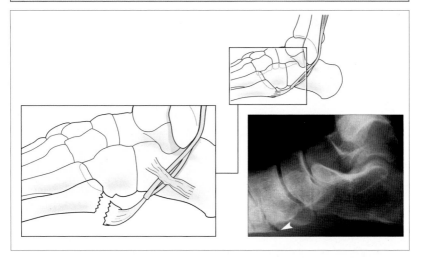

**Figure 13.23** *Inversion injury. The peroneus brevis tendon inserts into the base of the fifth metatarsal. An inversion force can cause an avulsion fracture. Lateral ankle showing fracture at base of fifth metatarsal (arrow)*

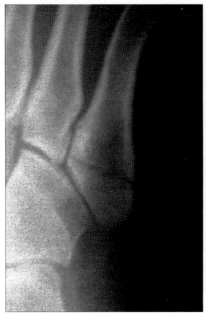

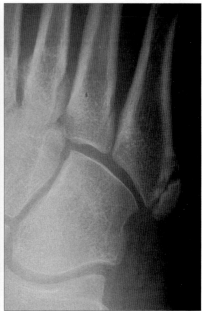

**Figure 13.24** *Fracture of the base of the fifth metatarsal. The fracture line is at right angles to the lateral cortex of the bone. This distinguishes it from a normal unfused apophysis.*

**Figure 13.25** *Typical appearance of an unfused apophysis at the base of the fifth metatarsal. The rule: the long axis of an apophysis tends to parallel the lateral cortex of the shaft of the metatarsal.*

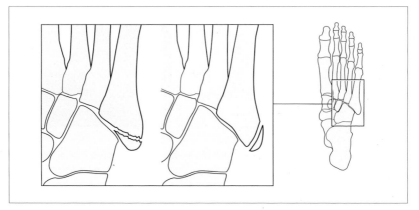

**Figure 13.26** *Typical appearances: an unfused apophysis (right) and a fracture (left) at the base of the fifth metatarsal.*

## LIGAMENTOUS INJURIES – AT THE MORTICE JOINT

■ If there is widening of one side of the joint space (Fig. 13.9) then there is commonly an associated fracture elsewhere

■ The radiographs may appear normal even when there is severe ligamentous damage. Sometimes stress views will be required/requested

■ A tear of the interosseous ligament is very easy to overlook.[3,5,8,9] The AP radiograph will often provide evidence of a tear/rupture:

❑ Look for widening of the space between the distal tibia and fibula

❑ A useful rule of thumb: suspect a tear if the distal tibia and fibula do not overlap slightly on the AP mortice view

❑ Apply the 6 mm rule (Fig. 13.5).

## KEY POINTS

- Apply the guideline: *no need for routine foot films when the ankle alone is injured*

- Careful clinical examination of the entire hindfoot and upper leg is essential. In addition to malleolar fractures and ligamentous injuries a twisted ankle may result in a fracture of:
  - ❏ the base of the fifth metatarsal
  - ❏ the upper fibula
  - ❏ the calcaneum

- An avulsion fracture at the base of the fifth metatarsal is common. A normal unfused apophysis should not be confused with a fracture fragment
  - ❏ **fracture**: the lucent line is transverse
  - ❏ **apophysis**: the lucent line is parallel to the long axis of the metatarsal.

## THE SUBTLE SIGN NOT TO MISS

- A small step or irregularity in the articular surface of the talar dome seen on the AP projection. The abnormality is most commonly situated on either the far medial or the far lateral aspect of the cortex

- These osteochondral fractures are often overlooked.

# REFERENCES

1. Stiell I, Wells G, Laupacis A *et al*. Multicentre trial to introduce the Ottawa ankle rules for use of radiography in acute ankle injuries. BMJ 1995; 311: 594–597.
2. Leddy JJ, Smolinski RJ, Lawrence J *et al*. Prospective evaluation of the Ottawa Ankle Rules in a University Sports Medicine Centre. AMJ Sports Med 1998; 26: 158–165.
3. Harper MC, Keller TS. A radiographic evaluation of the tibiofibular syndesmosis. Foot Ankle 1989; 10: 156–160.
4. Canale ST, Belding RH. Osteochondral lesions of the talus. J Bone Joint Surg AM 1980; 62: 97–102.
5. Brandser EA, Braksiek RJ, El-Khoury GY *et al*. Missed fractures on emergency room ankle radiographs: an analysis of 433 patients. Emergency Radiology 1997; 4: 295–302.
6. Prokuski LJ, Saltzman CL. Challenging fractures of the foot and ankle. Rad Clin North America 1997; 35: 655–670.
7. Slatis P, Kiviluoto O, Santavirta S *et al*. Fractures of the calcaneum. J Trauma 1979; 19: 939–943.
8. Ramsey PL, Hamilton W. Changes in tibiotalar area of contact caused by lateral talar shift. J Bone Joint Surg Am 1976; 58: 356–357.
9. Edwards GS, Delee JC. Ankle diastasis without fracture. Foot Ankle 1984; 4: 305–312.

# 14 MIDFOOT AND FOREFOOT

An injury to the midfoot or forefoot without appreciable/significant signs or symptoms can be treated without radiography.[1] An injury to a phalanx or to a metatarsal which will be treated by strapping – whether or not a fracture is present – does not need radiography.

## BASIC RADIOGRAPHS

- AP
- Oblique.

## ANATOMY

The bones of the midfoot form an arch. Consequently, several of the tarsal bones and the bases of the metatarsals (MT) overlap on both the AP and oblique projections. When the two views are assessed together the various bones can be separated.

### MIDFOOT ALIGNMENTS

The base of the second MT is held in a mortice created by the three cuneiform bones (Figs 14.1 and 14.2). This mortice arrangement prevents lateral slip of the bases of the metatarsals during weight bearing.

The normal tarsometatarsal alignments are as follows:

- The medial margin of the base of the **second** metatarsal should align with the medial margin of the intermediate cuneiform on the **AP view** (Figs 14.2, 14.3)
- The medial margin of the base of the **third** metatarsal should align with the medial margin of the lateral cuneiform on the **oblique view** (Figs 14.4, 14.5)

### MIDFOOT AND FOREFOOT ACCESSORY OSSICLES

These are numerous. They occasionally cause confusion (Fig. 1.8). Those ossicles which can mimic a fracture are illustrated in Keats' Atlas.[2]

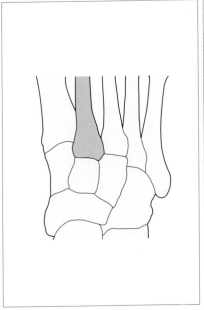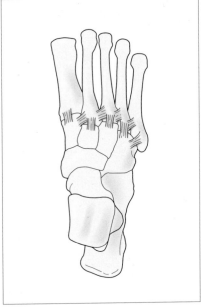

**Figure 14.1** *The base of the second metatarsal is held in the mortice created by the cuneiform bones. When weight bearing or walking it is this mortice and the strong surrounding ligaments which prevent lateral slippage of the bases of the metatarsals.*

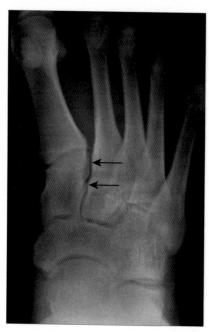

**Figure 14.2** *AP view. Normal. The medial margin of the second metatarsal is in line with the medial margin of the intermediate cuneiform bone (arrows).*

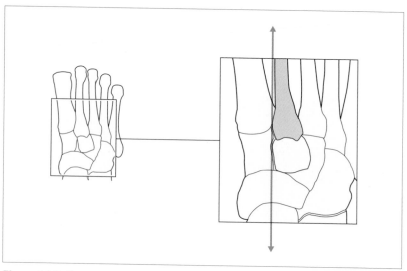

**Figure 14.3** *Normal alignment at the tarsometatarsal joints on the AP view.*

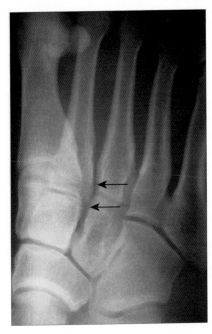

**Figure 14.4** *Oblique view. Normal. The medial margin of the third metatarsal (arrow) is in line with the medial margin of the lateral cuneiform (arrow). The base of the second metatarsal is partly obscured by overlapping bones.*

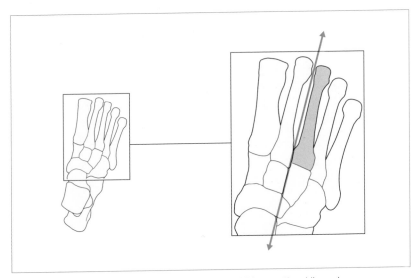

**Figure 14.5** *Normal alignment at the tarsometatarsal joints on the oblique view.*

## MIDFOOT FRACTURES AND DISLOCATIONS

### Tarsal fractures

Uncommon. Result from severe trauma. A major injury will be clinically obvious.

### Tarsometatarsal subluxations and dislocations

Important injuries.[3,4] Walking and weight-bearing depend on the accurate alignment of these bones. A dislocation or subluxation (Fig. 14.6) requires meticulous reduction in order to preserve/restore function.

■ Traumatic subluxations and dislocations at the bases of the metatarsals (Lisfranc injuries) will be overlooked unless the normal alignment of the bones (Figs 14.1–14.9) is carefully assessed. The radiographic appearance indicating a subluxation is often subtle. There are two questions to answer:

1. *On the AP view (Fig. 14.2) does the medial margin of the base of the second metatarsal align with the medial margin of the intermediate cuneiform?*

2. *On the oblique view (Fig. 14.4) does the medial margin of the third metatarsal align with the medial margin of the lateral cuneiform?*

■ When a fracture occurs through the second metatarsal distal to its base, the proximal fragment is held in place by the ligaments within the cuneiform mortice. The distal fragment then dislocates laterally together with the third, fourth and fifth metatarsals. In this circumstance it is the alignment of the medial margin of the third metatarsal with the medial margin of the lateral cuneiform that is disrupted (Fig. 14.7)

■ A tarso-metatarsal subluxation should be suspected whenever a fragment of bone is detached from the base of any of the medial four metatarsals.

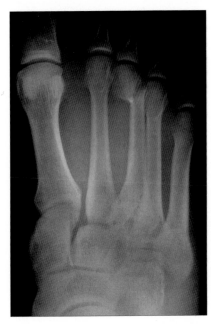

**Figure 14.6** *Injury to a Lisfranc joint. This is shown by the loss of the normal alignment at the base of the second metatarsal on this AP view. (Incidental fracture of the neck of the third metatarsal.)*

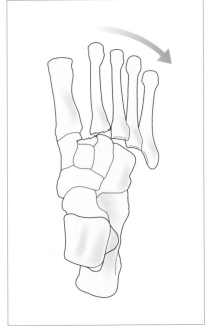

**Figure 14.7** *Fracture near the base of the second metatarsal frees the shaft of this bone from the cuneiform mortice. As a consequence, lateral slippage of the metatarsal bases has occurred.*

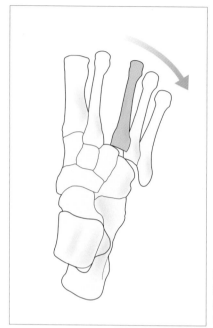

**Figure 14.8** *Lisfranc injury. Subluxation of the third, fourth and fifth metatarsals shown on the oblique view.*

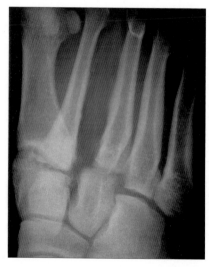

**Figure 14.9** *Injury to a Lisfranc (i.e. a tarsometatarsal) joint. This is shown by the loss of the normal alignment at the base of the third metatarsal on this oblique view.*

# FOREFOOT FRACTURES

## The fifth metatarsal

*Avulsion fracture of the tuberosity*
A fracture of the tuberosity at the base of this metatarsal is described in detail on page 231. It is worth restating a few aspects:

- A fracture of the tuberosity represents an avulsion injury resulting from contraction of the peroneus brevis muscle. It is caused by a plantar flexion – inversion injury[3]

- Careful clinical examination of the base of the metatarsal will indicate that radiography of the foot, not the ankle, is necessary

- This fracture can be treated as for weight-bearing – with strapping or a walking plaster

- The normal unfused apophysis at the base of the fifth metatarsal is present in all children (see page 232). It should not be misinterpreted as a fracture.

*The Jones' fracture[4–7]*
Occurs as either an acute injury or as a fatigue fracture. It is often confused with a fracture of the tuberosity.

- It does not result from an avulsion injury

- The fracture is sited in the diaphysis within 1.5 cm of the tuberosity (Fig. 14.10). Relevant features: a Jones' fracture lies distal to both the tarso-metatarsal joint and to the joint between the fourth and fifth metatarsals

- An important injury. Non-union is common. Treatment with a non-weight-bearing cast is necessary. In elite athletes fixation with an intramedullary screw is often required.

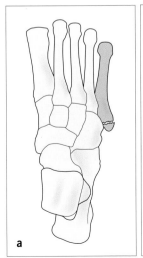

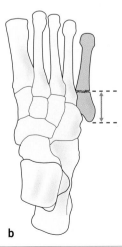

**Figure 14.10** *Fractures involving the proximal third of the fifth metatarsal. Different mechanisms and differing prognosis. (a) A typical avulsion fracture of the tuberosity. Prognosis is excellent. (b) A Jones' fracture is positioned in the diaphysis within 1.5 cm of the tip of the tuberosity. Not an avulsion injury. There are acute and chronic (stress) Jones' fractures. Non-union is a relatively common complication.*

a          b

### Fatigue (march/stress) fractures

These injuries are frequently missed, misdiagnosed, mistreated, and misunderstood.[5]

- The second and third metatarsal shafts are most commonly affected

- Radiographs are only abnormal when the fracture is well established (Fig. 14.11)

- Four radiographic patterns:

  - ❏ Normal radiograph

  - ❏ Transverse crack

  - ❏ Faint periosteal reaction or fluffy callus

  - ❏ Profuse callus

- If clinical suspicion of a fatigue fracture is high and the initial radiographs appear normal, then it is worth considering a radionuclide bone study. Localised increase in uptake of the radiopharmaceutical in the context of a relevant history is diagnostic of a fatigue fracture.[5]

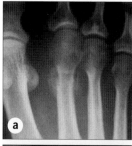
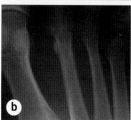
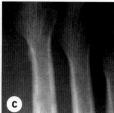
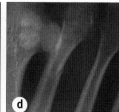

**Figure 14.11** *Stress fractures. Four different patients. (a) Periosteal new bone is easy to see. (b, c) Periosteal new bone formation is more subtle. (d) The fracture is seen as a lucent line only.*

## KEY POINTS

### Midfoot

■ A Lisfranc midfoot subluxation or dislocation may be subtle. Check whether the anatomy is normal by confirming that:

❑ The medial margin of the base of the second metatarsal lines up with the medial margin of the intermediate cuneiform on the AP view

❑ The medial margin of the base of the third metatarsal lines up with the medial margin of the lateral cuneiform on the oblique view.

### Forefoot

■ An avulsion fracture of the tuberosity at the base of the fifth metatarsal is common and results from inversion of the ankle

■ When pain is chronic, or there has been no single episode of acute trauma, consider the diagnosis of a metatarsal fatigue fracture, particularly in an adolescent or a young adult.

## THE SUBTLE SIGN NOT TO MISS

■ A bone fragment is detached from the base of any one of the first four metatarsals. A tarsometatarsal subluxation should be suspected/excluded

■ Subluxation is serious. Weight bearing and walking is dependent on accurate alignment at the tarsometatarsal (i.e. the Lisfranc) joint.

## REFERENCES

1. David HG. Value of radiographs in managing common foot injuries. Br Med J 1989; 298: 1491–1492.
2. Keats TE. Atlas of normal roentgen variants that may simulate disease, 7th ed. Year Book Medical Publishers, Chicago, 2001.
3. Anderson LD. Injuries of the forefoot. Clin Orthopaed Rel Res 1977; 122: 18–27.
4. Prokuski LJ, Saltzman CL. Challenging fractures of the foot and ankle. Rad Clin North Am 1997; 35: 655–670.
5. Anderson EG. Fatigue fractures of the foot. Injury 1990; 21: 275–279.
6. Berquist TH. Radiology of the foot and ankle, 2nd ed. Philadelphia, PA: Lippincott Williams and Wilkins, 2000.
7. Lawrence SJ, Botte MJ. Jones' fractures and related fractures of the proximal fifth metatarsal. Foot Ankle 1993; 14: 358–365.
8. Inokuchi S, Usami N. Jones' fracture. The Foot 1997; 7: 75–78.

# 15 CHEST

- The chest radiograph (CXR) is the most frequently requested radiological investigation in the Emergency Department (ED). It is an essential clinical tool. For example, physical examination is not sufficiently accurate on its own to confirm or exclude the diagnosis of pneumonia[1]

- Although the full scope of the radiology of thoracic emergencies[2–7] needs the space provided by a larger textbook, in practice *10 clinical questions account for over 90% of CXR requests made in the ED*.

## BASIC RADIOGRAPHY

- If possible: a PA erect CXR in full inspiration

- Severely ill patient: an AP radiograph in the semi-erect or supine position

- On occasion, a lateral CXR can be useful when seeking to confirm or clarify an abnormality shown on the frontal projection.

## NORMAL APPEARANCES AND IMPORTANT ANATOMY

### GENERAL
### On the frontal chest radiograph (Fig. 15.1)
These rules apply to both PA and AP projections:

- The left and right heart borders are well defined

- Both domes of the diaphragm* are visible to the midline

- A good inspiration is desirable. A small inspiration can produce misleading appearances (Fig. 15.2), including:

  ❏ Spurious cardiac enlargement

  ❏ Increased basal shadowing due to crowding of vessels. This can mimic lung consolidation or oedema.

---

* The word 'diaphragms' is incorrect. Only one diaphragm separates the chest from the abdomen. It has two domes.

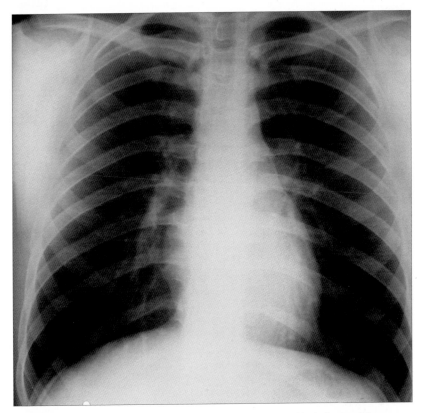

**Figure 15.1** *Normal PA chest radiograph. Both heart borders and both domes of the diaphragm are sharp and well defined.*

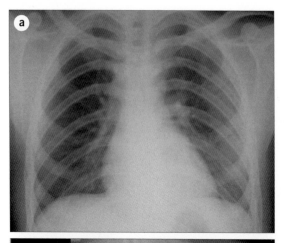

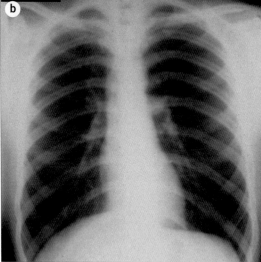

**Figure 15.2** *Effects of a poor inspiration (a). The transverse cardiac diameter exceeds 50% of the diameter of the chest and raises the possibility of cardiac enlargement. Also, both lungs show areas of increased density at the bases. The film was repeated a few minutes later following a full inspiration (b). The transverse cardiac diameter is now normal and the lungs are clear.*

## On the lateral chest radiograph[8–10]

- One dome of the diaphragm (the right) is visible from the anterior chest wall to the posterior costophrenic recess (Fig. 15.3)

- The other dome (the left) is only visible from the posterior aspect of the cardiac shadow to the posterior costophrenic recess

- The lower thoracic vertebral bodies appear darker compared with the vertebrae in the mid and upper thorax – because the overlying soft tissues of the chest wall and axillae are denser at the higher levels.

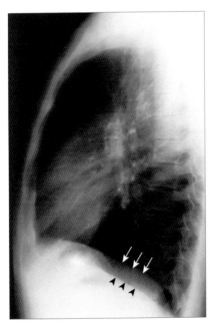

**Figure 15.3** *Normal lateral chest radiograph. Note that both hemidiaphragms are seen (arrows, right dome; arrowheads, left dome) and that the lower thoracic vertebral bodies appear darker than those in the mid and upper thorax.*

## HILA

- The hilum is the site at which the bronchi and vessels enter/leave the lung. On a CXR, the hilar shadow is composed mainly of the pulmonary artery and veins (Fig. 15.4)

- The left pulmonary artery passes over the left main bronchus, whereas the right pulmonary artery passes in front of the main bronchus. This is why the left hilum is higher than the right hilum on the CXR

- The rule to apply: *if the left hilum appears to be lower than the right then an abnormality, on one side or the other, should always be suspected*

- Occasionally, a hilum is difficult to assess. Is it low/high/enlarged or normal vessels only? In practice, accurate analysis of an equivocal appearance requires the opinion of an experienced observer.

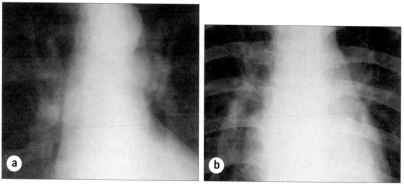

**Figure 15.4** *Normal hila in two different patients. Hilar shadows are mainly due to pulmonary vessels. In most patients the left hilum is higher than the right (a). In a few normal patients the hila are at the same level (b). The rule to apply:* **on the normal CXR the left hilum is never lower than the right hilum**.

## HEART

- **Cardiac enlargement.** A useful rule of thumb: *most normal hearts have a cardiothoracic ratio (CTR) of less than 50% when assessed on a PA chest radiograph obtained in full inspiration*[11]

- **Measuring the CTR** (Fig. 15.5). Two lines are drawn tangential to the outermost aspects of the right and left sides of the heart. The transverse diameter of the thorax is measured as the maximum *internal* width of the thoracic cage (i.e. rib to rib).

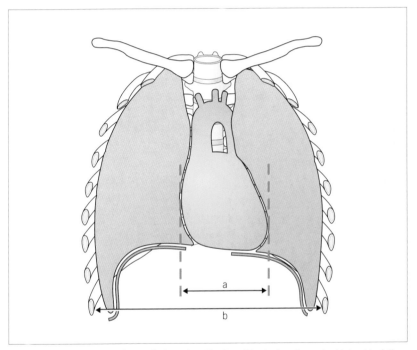

**Figure 15.5** *Measuring the cardiothoracic ratio. On a PA chest radiograph obtained in full inspiration, if a/b > 50% the heart is likely to be enlarged.[11] a = maximum transverse diameter of the heart; b = maximum internal diameter of the thorax.*

## CONSOLIDATION

Where lung alveoli fill with fluid there will be a density on the radiograph... consolidation. Although the word 'consolidation' is often used synonymously with infective pneunomia there are other causes of this air space shadowing. These include: pulmonary haemorrhage, oedema and aspiration.

## TEN QUESTIONS ... ACCOUNTING FOR 90% OF CXR REQUESTS IN THE EMERGENCY DEPARTMENT

### QUESTION 1

#### Is there a cause for non-specific chest pain?

- In many of these patients the pain remains unexplained and the CXR is normal

- Note: following an acute myocardial infarction the CXR may be entirely normal. Sometimes the heart will be enlarged.

### QUESTION 2

#### Is there pneumonia (consolidation)?

- Malaise, cough, and fever but few other signs or symptoms is a common presentation – pneumonia needs to be excluded

- Clinical examination alone is unreliable.[1] Physical examination has a sensitivity of about 50%; the specificity is not much better – as low as 58%

- Many pneumonias will be obvious on the frontal CXR. Some are more difficult to detect – the concealed consolidation.

#### Rules for detecting concealed consolidation

- Assess the mediastinal and diaphragmatic boundaries (Fig. 15.1) by answering this question: *'are both heart borders and both domes of the diaphragm well defined and clearly visible?'*

- The principle: the borders of the heart and both domes of the diaphragm are visible on a normal CXR because the air in the lung contrasts with the water density of the heart and diaphragm (see Fig. 1.1). If lung air is replaced by pus (pneumonia) the immediately adjacent border will disappear or be ill-defined

- When a border is ill-defined, the precise site of a concealed area of consolidation can be deduced (Table 15.1). Sometimes loss of a border is more obvious than the air space density, particularly when there is accompanying volume loss (collapse) of the affected lobe or segment (Figs 15.9, 15.10).

**Table 15.1** Pneumonia – borders to check

| Ill defined or absent | Suspect consolidation and/or collapse of the |
|---|---|
| Right heart border | Middle lobe |
| Left heart border | Upper lobe |
| Right dome of diaphragm | Lower lobe |
| Left dome of diaphragm | Lower lobe |

See examples in Figs 15.6–15.11.

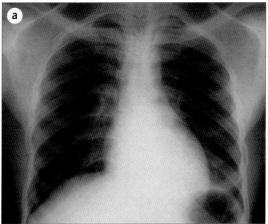

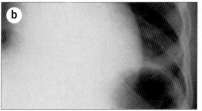

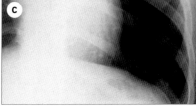

**Figure 15.6** *Left lower lobe consolidation (with some collapse). The medial aspect of the left hemidiaphragm is not sharply defined (a, b). After treatment for pneumonia the normal appearance of the diaphragm is shown in (c).*

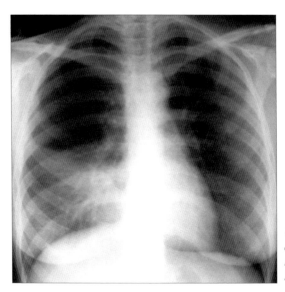

**Figure 15.7** *Middle lobe consolidation. The right heart border is ill defined and there is an adjacent density.*

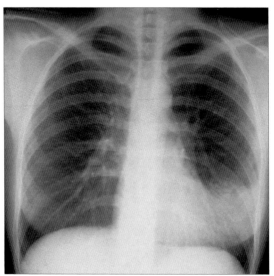

**Figure 15.8** *Left upper lobe consolidation. Increased shadowing in the lower zone of the left lung. The lower part of the left heart border is ill defined, indicating that the consolidation is in the inferior segment of the lingula. (The lingula corresponds to the middle lobe of the right lung but anatomically it is part of the left upper lobe.)*

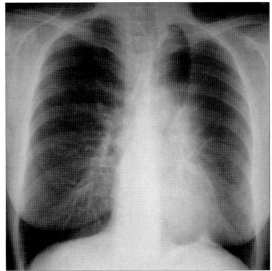

**Figure 15.9** *Left upper lobe collapse. The entire left heart border is ill defined. This indicates an abnormality of the upper lobe. The ill-defined border is more obvious than any added density. The well-defined lucency overlying the medial aspect of the upper zone represents part of the right lung herniating across the midline. This combination of findings is characteristic of a collapse of the entire left upper lobe.*

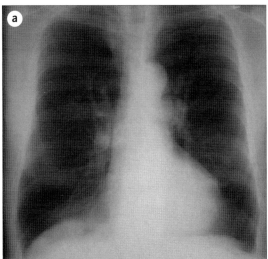

**Figure 15.10** *Right lower lobe consolidation with some collapse. Shadowing in the lower zone of the right lung (a, b). The medial part of the right dome of the diaphragm is not sharply defined, indicating that the consolidation is in the lower lobe. The normal appearance of the diaphragm after treatment is shown in (c).*

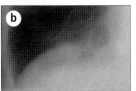

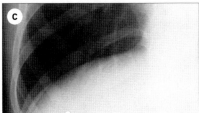

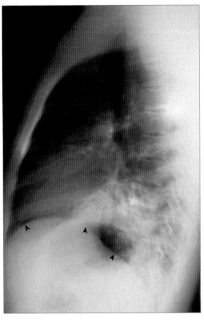

**Figure 15.11** *Two abnormalities on this lateral CXR indicate that there is consolidation in the left lower lobe. (1) Only one dome of the diaphragm is visualised – i.e. the upper surface of the right dome (arrowheads). The left dome is not seen. (2) The lower vertebral bodies appear more opaque (denser/whiter) than those in the upper thorax. Compare with a normal lateral CXR (Fig. 15.3).*

## QUESTION 3

### Is there a pneumothorax?

■ A PA CXR obtained in full expiration is recommended. The normal lungs are more opaque on an expiration CXR. Consequently, when a pneumothorax is present the air (black) in the pleural space contrasts with the adjacent (whiter) lung. This accentuation of the difference in contrast as compared with an inspiration film makes it easier to detect a pneumothorax

■ A pneumothorax shows three features on the erect CXR:

❑ A clearly defined line (i.e. the visceral pleura) – this line parallels the chest wall (Fig. 15.12)

❑ The upper part of this line will be curved at the lung apex

❑ An absence of lung markings (i.e. vessels) between the lung edge and the chest wall.

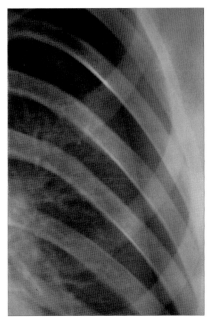

**Figure 15.12**
*Pneumothorax. Note the
well-defined line that represents
the lung edge (i.e. the visceral
pleura). Also, there are no
vessels lateral to this line.*

## QUESTION 4

### Severe asthmatic attack – is there a complication?

The complications to look for are:

- Lung consolidation

- Lobar collapse

- Pneumothorax

- Pneumomediastinum – streaks of air in the mediastinal soft tissues.
  These streaks may extend up into the neck. (Often this is a subtle finding only
  detectable by an experienced observer.)

## QUESTION 5

### Are there features of left ventricular failure (i.e. pulmonary venous hypertension)?

**Look for:**

**1.** *Cardiac enlargement*

■ Almost all patients with left ventricular failure (LVF) have cardiomegaly. The occasional exception is a patient with an acute myocardial infarction

■ Most enlarged hearts have a CTR over 50% when assessed on a PA CXR (Fig. 15.5).

---

## Pitfalls

■ A CTR measurement is not valid:

  ❏ On an AP CXR – because of magnification

  ❏ In some elderly patients when the internal thoracic diameter is reduced because of bone (rib) softening

  ❏ When the sternum is depressed – a depressed sternum or a very narrow AP diameter of the thorax can cause the CTR to exceed 50%

■ A few normal people (approximately 2%)[11] have a CTR over 50%

■ A heart may be enlarged despite a normal CTR – the transverse cardiac diameter might have been very narrow when the heart was normal and the enlargement has not yet reached 50% of the transverse diameter of the thorax.

---

**2.** *Changes in the calibre of the pulmonary vessels*

■ When the pulmonary venous pressure is normal the upper lobe vessels are smaller in diameter than the lower lobe vessels on the erect CXR

■ As the venous pressure begins to rise these diameters are reversed as the upper lobe vessels enlarge and the lower lobe vessels constrict (Fig. 15.13)

■ This radiological appearance of upper lobe blood diversion is very, very subtle, and is often erroneously claimed/stated in order to fit the clinical picture and other more reliable radiological signs (see Glossary: Emperor's new clothes).

**3.** *Lung and pleural changes*

■ A wide spectrum of changes occurs as the venous pressure rises even further (Table 15.2)

■ The precise changes will vary between individuals (Figs 15.13–15.19).

**Table 15.2** Left ventricular failure – signs on the erect CXR

| | |
|---|---|
| **Early** | Enlarged heart |
| | Upper lobe vessels are of wider diameter than lower lobe vessels |
| | Oedema: poorly defined (slightly blurred) margins of the hilar vessels |
| | Oedema: septal lines (Kerley B lines) |
| | Small pleural effusions – usually bilateral |
| **Later** | Interstitial shadowing (oedema) **and/or** |
| | Alveolar shadowing (florid oedema) **and/or** |
| | Pleural effusions of increasing size – usually bilateral |

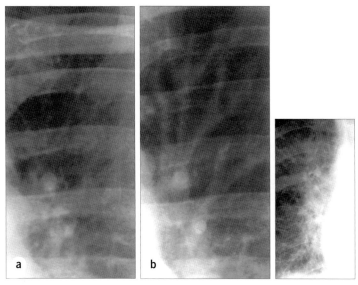

a  b

**Figure 15.13** *Early LVF. Change in size of the upper lobe vessels when the pulmonary venous pressure was normal (a) and prior to developing florid pulmonary oedema (b). The upper lobe vessels are dilated in (b) as compared with (a). (This example is provided to illustrate that changes in vessel size do occur. Nevertheless, it is emphasised that evaluation of vessel size in early pulmonary venous hypertension can be very, very difficult.)*

**Figure 15.14** *Early LVF. Poorly defined margins of the hilar vessels due to perivascular oedema.*

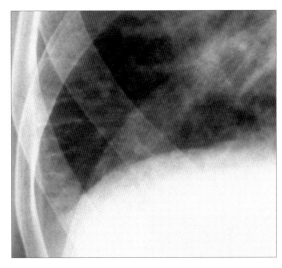

**Figure 15.15** *Early LVF. Septal lines (Kerley B lines) caused by fluid in the interstitium. These short, straight lines reach the pleural surface and have this characteristic appearance.*

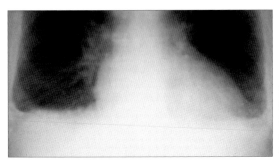

**Figure 15.16** *Early LVF. Small pleural effusions. Slight blunting of the costophrenic angles. Effusions in LVF are usually bilateral.*

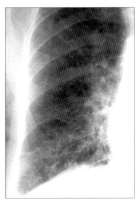

**Figure 15.17** *Florid LVF. Extensive interstitial oedema. The fluid lies mainly in the interstitium of the lung.*

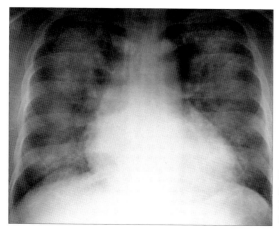

**Figure 15.18** *Florid LVF. Extensive alveolar oedema. The alveolar air spaces have filled with fluid.*

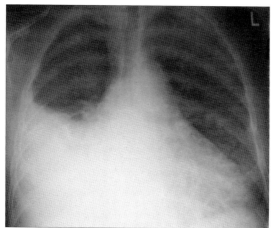

**Figure 15.19** *Florid LVF. The main finding is a large pleural effusion. When pleural effusions occur they are usually bilateral. Unilateral effusions are most often situated on the right side.*

## QUESTION 6

### Is there a pleural effusion?

There are numerous causes for a pleural effusion. Also, fluid in the pleural space can adopt several different appearances on the CXR.

### On the erect frontal CXR

■ The commonest appearance is a meniscus at a costophrenic angle. It requires approximately 200 ml of pleural fluid to efface the normal sharp sulcus between the diaphragm and the ribs (Fig. 15.20). If the effusion is large, the entire hemithorax is opaque and the heart is pushed towards the normal side (Fig. 15.20)

■ There are other patterns:

❏ A linear (lamellar) shadow paralleling the lateral aspect of the lung (Fig. 15.21)

❏ Loculation within a fissure (Fig. 15.22)

❏ Puddling in a subpulmonary position (Figs 15.23, 15.24). This is a relatively common occurrence. A subpulmonary effusion is usually easier to detect on the left side, where the puddle in the pleural space can cause the gastric air bubble to appear widely separate from the (apparent) superior margin of the diaphragm (Fig. 15.24).

### On the supine CXR

Approximately 200 ml of fluid must be present before abnormal shadowing is produced.[12,13] The shadowing is seen as an increase in density of the affected hemithorax (Fig. 15.25). The fluid layers out in the posterior pleural space and this causes the hemithorax to appear greyer or whiter than the other side. In most instances the normal lung vessels will be seen through this shadowing.

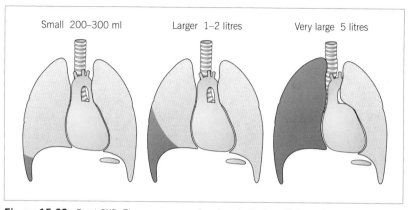

**Figure 15.20** *Erect CXR. The appearance of a pleural effusion will depend on its size.*

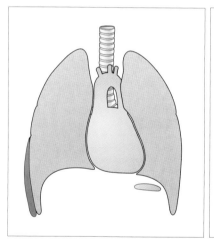

**Figure 15.21** *An occasional appearance: a lamellar pleural effusion. The fluid parallels the lateral margin and the sharp costophrenic sulcus is preserved.*

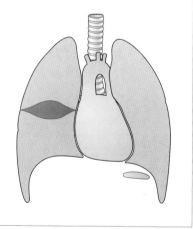

**Figure 15.22** *An occasional appearance: fluid encysted within a fissure. In this example, the fluid has collected within the horizontal fissure.*

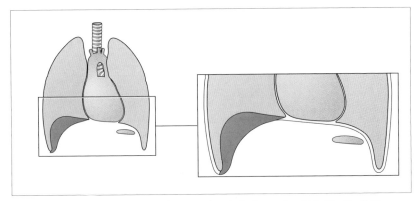

**Figure 15.23** *Erect CXR. A subpulmonary pleural effusion on the right side. The fluid (the black area) collects between the visceral and parietal pleura at the base of the lung. The effect on the erect CXR is to simulate an elevated dome of the diaphragm.*

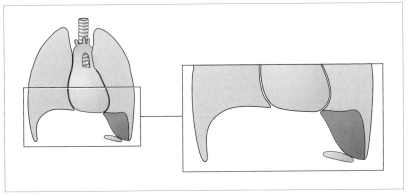

**Figure 15.24** *Erect CXR. A subpulmonary pleural effusion on the left side. The fluid (the black area) has pooled between the visceral and parietal pleura at the base of the lung. The net effect on the erect CXR is to simulate an elevated dome of the diaphragm. A clue to the presence of a subpulmonary effusion on the left side is the low position of the gastric air bubble.*

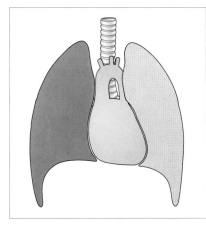

**Figure 15.25** *Supine CXR. A right-sided effusion has spread out posteriorly within the pleural space. This produces a slightly more opaque hemithorax when compared with the normal side.*

## QUESTION 7

### Is there evidence of a pulmonary embolus?[14]

- 90% of emboli occur without pulmonary infarction

  - The CXR appearance is often normal

  - Sometimes non-specific findings are present: small areas of linear collapse and/or a small pleural effusion and/or slight elevation of a dome of the diaphragm

  - Unilateral lucency (i.e. hypertransradiancy) due to an area of reduced perfusion does occur but it is a very rare finding

- 10% of emboli present with pulmonary infarction

  - The CXR appearances are variable – similar to an embolus without infarction (see above)

  - An area of consolidation

  - A pleural effusion

  - Consolidation and an effusion

- The CXR may reveal an unexpected and definitive cause for chest pain in a patient clinically suspected of a pulmonary embolus (e.g. a pneumothorax). When a pulmonary embolus remains a clinical possibility then – whatever the CXR findings (lung consolidation or non-specific changes) – the patient requires definitive imaging, either a radionuclide study or a CT pulmonary angiogram.

## QUESTION 8

### Is there an aortic dissection or traumatic rupture of the aorta?

When assessing the mediastinum there are no absolute measurements that indicate abnormal widening. In middle-aged and elderly patients the aorta will often show age-related unfolding (Fig. 15.26). On an AP projection an unfolded but otherwise normal aorta can be considerably magnified.

## AORTIC DISSECTION[14]

■ The CXR is often normal

■ In the appropriate clinical setting mediastinal widening (Fig. 15.26), with or without a left pleural effusion, is highly suggestive

■ Clinical suspicion of a dissection must take priority over a normal CXR.

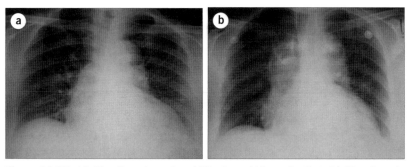

**Figure 15.26** *(a) AP radiograph: aortic unfolding in a middle-aged patient. (b) AP radiograph: the same patient presenting a few years later to the Emergency Department. Widening of the mediastinum has increased due to a dissection. Investigation of a dissection depends upon the history and clinical examination rather than the plain film appearance.*

## TRAUMATIC RUPTURE[4,5,7]

■ 30% of patients have a normal CXR on presentation

■ A widened mediastinum does not necessarily indicate aortic rupture. Tearing of small mediastinal veins is the most common cause of mediastinal widening following a high-impact collision

■ Clinical concern will determine the need for a definitive radiographic examination (e.g. CT).

## QUESTION 9

### Is there a rib fracture?

Oblique views of the ribs are not indicated following a relatively minor injury to the thorax. Clinical management is rarely altered by the demonstration of a simple rib fracture. A frontal CXR is obtained solely to exclude an important complication such as a pneumothorax.

## QUESTION 10

### Is there evidence of an inhaled foreign body?

See page 324 in Chapter 19.

## KEY POINTS

■ Pneumonia – both heart borders and both domes of the diaphragm should be clearly visible. Loss of clarity raises the probability of adjacent lung consolidation or collapse

■ Pulmonary embolism – the CXR can appear normal

■ Cardiac enlargement is likely when the CTR is over 50% on a PA CXR

■ Left heart failure can be a difficult clinical diagnosis in breathless elderly patients. The CXR may make the diagnosis obvious

■ Pneumothorax – most easily seen on an expiration CXR

■ An unfolded aorta can be considerably magnified on an AP CXR. Aortic dissection or rupture may be erroneously attributed to age-related aortic unfolding. Clinical findings determine the need for additional imaging

■ Simple rib fracture – oblique films not indicated.

## THE SUBTLE SIGN NOT TO MISS

| Clinical history | Supine CXR | Explanation |
|---|---|---|
| Road traffic accident: injured right side of chest | Rib fractures (right), a shallow pneumothorax **and** *the right hemithorax also appears uniformly grey compared with the left side; lung vessels are readily identified through the greyness* | ■ Not a simple pneumothorax<br>■ Blood in the pleural space – the fluid has layered out posteriorly and causes the grey appearance<br>■ Diagnosis: *a haemopneumothorax* |

# REFERENCES

1. Wipf JE, Lipsky BA, Hirschmann JV. Diagnosing pneumonia by physical examination. Relevant or relic? Arch Intern Med 1999; 159: 1082–1087.
2. Armstrong P, Wilson AG, Dee P, Hansell DM. Imaging of diseases of the chest. St Louis, MO: Mosby, 2000.
3. Armstrong P. Chest. In: Keats TE, ed. Emergency radiology, 2nd ed. Chicago, IL: Year Book; 1989.
4. Schnyder P, Wintermark M. Radiology of blunt trauma of the chest. Berlin: Springer-Verlag, 2000.
5. Mirvis SE, Templeton P. Imaging in acute thoracic trauma. Semin Roentgenol 1992; 27: 84–210.
6. Groskin SA. Selected topics in chest trauma. Radiology 1992; 183: 605–617.
7. Gavelli G, Canini R, Bertaccini P et al. Traumatic injuries: imaging of thoracic injuries. Eur Radiol 2002; 12: 1273–1294.
8. Austin JHM. The lateral chest radiograph in the assessment of non-pulmonary health and disease. RCNA 1984; 22: 687–698.
9. Whalen JP, Lane EF. Bronchial re-arrangements in pulmonary collapse as seen on the lateral radiograph. Radiology 1969; 93: 285–288.
10. Vix VA, Klatte EC. The lateral chest radiograph in the diagnosis of hilar and mediastinal masses. Radiology 1970; 96: 307–316.
11. Felson B. Chest roentgenology. Philadelphia, PA: WB Saunders, 1973: 496.
12. Emamian SA, Kaasbol MA, Olsen JF et al. Accuracy of the diagnosis of pleural effusion on supine chest X-ray. Eur Radiol 1997; 7: 57–60.
13. Woodring JH. Recognition of pleural effusion on supine radiographs: how much fluid is required? AJR 1984; 142: 59–64.
14. Reed JC. Chest radiology: plain film patterns and differential diagnosis. 5th ed. St Louis, MO: Mosby, 2003.

# 16 ABDOMEN

## ACUTE ABDOMINAL PAIN ... NO TRAUMA

### INDICATIONS FOR PLAIN ABDOMINAL RADIOGRAPHY

- Plain abdominal radiography (AXR) is indicated[1-3] for suspected:
  - Perforation – supine AXR and erect chest (CXR)
  - Obstruction – supine AXR and erect CXR
  - Renal colic – supine AXR as part of a limited IVU series
- Ultrasound should be the first imaging procedure in:
  - Suspected biliary disease
  - Suspected abdominal aortic aneurysm/rupture
- CT is replacing some or all of the above studies in many centres.

## RADIOGRAPHIC TECHNIQUE AND FINDINGS

### SUSPECTED PERFORATION

- The most useful routine radiograph is a well-penetrated erect CXR (Fig. 16.1). If a patient is unable to sit up, an AXR is obtained in the left-side-down decubitus position using a horizontal X-ray beam (Fig. 16.2)
- Very small quantities (as little as 1.0 ml) of free air can be demonstrated.[4]

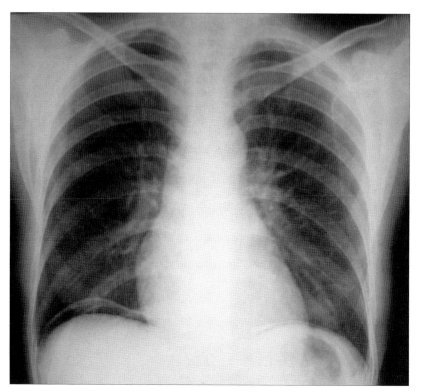

**Figure 16.1** *Perforation. Air is present under both domes of the diaphragm. A well-penetrated erect chest film is the single most useful radiograph for the demonstration of free intraperitoneal air.*

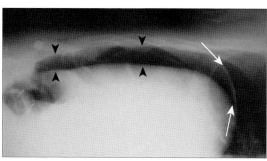

**Figure 16.2** *Perforation. Patient too unwell to sit up. A lateral decubitus film with the patient lying on the left side. A large amount of free intraperitoneal air is shown (between arrowheads) above the lateral surface of the liver. The air outlines the undersurface of the right dome of the diaphragm (arrows).*

## SUSPECTED INTESTINAL OBSTRUCTION

- Radiography: erect CXR and supine AXR[3,5]

- The CXR may reveal intrathoracic disease. Pneumonia can present as acute abdominal pain

- Some centres regard an erect AXR as unnecessary, arguing that it rarely adds any additional information to the supine film.[3,5] Others obtain an erect AXR since it may be useful in demonstrating:

  - Multiple small bowel fluid levels when the supine film shows relatively little evidence of small bowel distension. Multiple fluid levels and no gas distension can occur when a mechanical obstruction is present

  - The 'string of beads' sign (see below).

### Interpretation – some basic rules[6]

- *Dilated small bowel with an absence of colon gas* suggests a complete, or nearly complete, mechanical obstruction to the small bowel (Fig. 16.3)

- *Dilated small bowel with gas in an undistended colon* suggests **either**

  - An incomplete, mechanical, obstruction to the small bowel, **or**

  - A localized adynamic (i.e. paralytic) ileus

- *Dilated small bowel with gas in a distended colon* indicates **either**

  - A mechanical obstruction to the large bowel with an incompetent ileo-caecal valve, **or**

  - A generalised adynamic ileus (Fig. 16.5)

- *The 'string of beads sign'* invariably indicates a mechanical obstruction to the small bowel.[6] This sign is only seen on an AXR taken in the erect position (Fig. 16.6). The sign:

  - Occurs when dilated small bowel loops are almost completely filled with fluid and small bubbles of gas – a 'string of beads' – are trapped in the folds along the superior wall of the distended intestine

  - Is rarely seen in a patient with an adynamic (i.e. paralytic) ileus because there is usually only a small amount of fluid in the small bowel

- *Dilated large bowel but no small bowel dilatation* suggests mechanical obstruction to the large bowel with a competent ileocaecal valve (Fig. 16.4)

- *Dilated large bowel with dilated small bowel* suggests *either* mechanical large bowel obstruction with an incompetent ileocaecal valve *or* a generalised adynamic (i.e. paralytic) ileus (Fig. 16.5). The distinction is usually clinically obvious.

## Changing practice

- Some departments are using CT to assess suspected intestinal obstruction[1,7,8]

- The most sensible/appropriate algorithm for deciding between an AXR and CT is being evaluated/determined.[1]

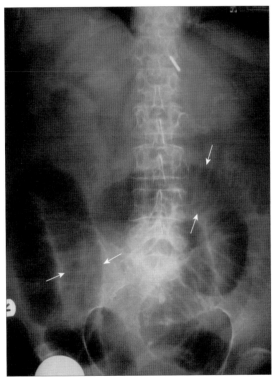

**Figure 16.3** *Colicky abdominal pain. Dilated loops of small bowel (arrows). Some loops measure 50 mm in diameter (whereas the upper limit of normal is 30 mm). Almost no gas within the large bowel. Mechanical small bowel obstruction.*

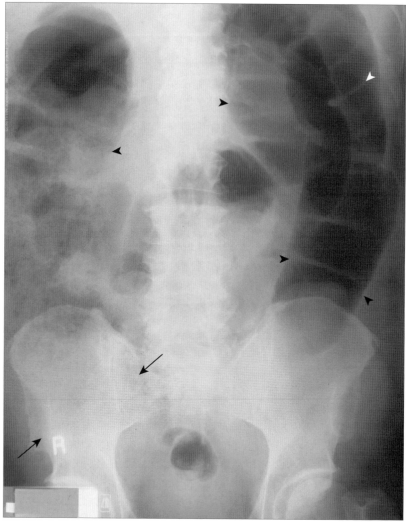

**Figure 16.4** *Colicky abdominal pain. Transverse colon and descending colon are dilated (arrowheads). A small amount of gas in the distal sigmoid. The caecum and ascending colon are also distended and contain faecal residue (arrows). These findings indicate a high grade mechanical obstruction in the distal descending colon or in the sigmoid colon. The absence of small bowel dilatation is due to a competent ileo-caecal valve. If the obstruction persists, then the small bowel will eventually become distended with gas.*

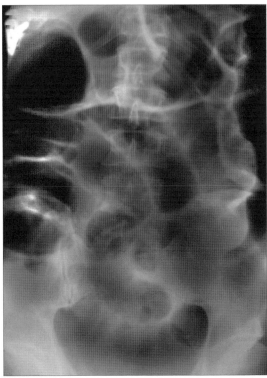

**Figure 16.5** *Generalised adynamic (i.e. paralytic) ileus. Centrally situated dilated loops of small bowel. The entire large bowel is also dilated. A similar pattern might be seen in a patient with a mechanical obstruction in the distal sigmoid colon. The clinical history will usually distinguish between these two possibilities.*

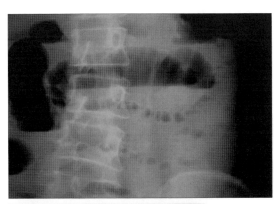

**Figure 16.6** *Erect AXR. 'String of beads' sign (i.e. small pockets of gas in a row). These 'beads' represent small amounts of gas caught between the mucosal folds of dilated small bowel distended mainly by fluid. Very little gaseous distension. This sign is only seen on an erect film and is virtually pathognomic of mechanical small bowel obstruction.*[6]

## SUSPECTED RENAL COLIC

■ An AXR is diagnostic when there is an obvious opaque calculus in the line of the renal tract. It is less helpful if the film appears normal. A calculus may be obscured by superimposed bone, may be confused with a pelvic phlebolith or may not be radio-opaque. Although 90% of renal calculi contain calcium, less than 50% are visible on an AXR.[9] A limited intravenous urogram (IVU) is highly accurate in confirming or excluding a calculus (Fig. 16.7)

■ There is now a trend to replace the limited IVU with a spiral CT examination (Fig. 16.8). Local preference will apply.[9]

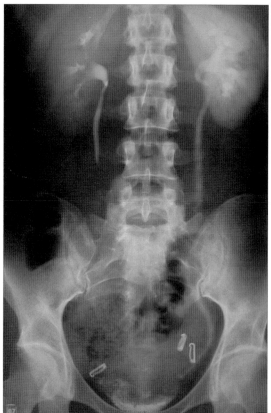

**Figure 16.7** *Clinical suspicion: acute left-sided ureteric colic. Feint calcification was seen in the true pelvis on the supine abdominal radiograph. A single film obtained 20 minutes after the injection of contrast medium confirms that a calculus is causing left-sided ureteric obstruction.*

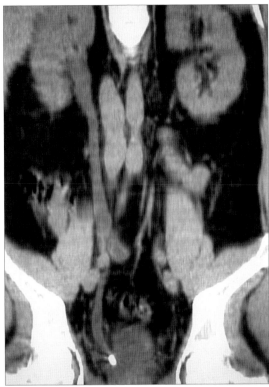

**Figure 16.8** *Clinical suspicion: acute right-sided ureteric colic. The patient was referred directly for a CT examination. The obstructing calculus at the vesico-ureteric junction was demonstrated – elegantly shown on this coronal reconstruction.*
*In many centres a CT examination is replacing the standard one-film IVU.*

**Pitfall:** Some centres use a combination of plain film and ultrasound examination to replace an IVU. This approach might appear logical but caution is advised. Because:

■ Ultrasound has a false negative rate as high as 30% in acute renal colic. The error rate is highest when ultrasound is performed shortly after the onset of symptoms[10]

■ If the ultrasound examination is normal, then a limited IVU (or CT) will still be necessary.

## PENETRATING INJURY OR BLUNT TRAUMA

In patients who have sustained abdominal or pelvic trauma the rapid assessment of injury is critical. Delay increases mortality and morbidity.[11]

■ Plain abdominal radiography is not indicated when investigating a blunt or penetrating injury – unless a retained metallic foreign body (e.g. bullet or blade) is suspected

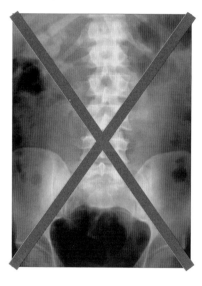

■ A description of the abnormal findings on plain AXR, essentially an outdated investigation, is not useful. Obtaining an AXR is strongly discouraged – it delays the useful investigations.

■ Recommendations in relation to imaging a **haemodynamically stable patient**:

  ❑ The unequivocal demonstration of a haemoperitoneum that is increasing in size will determine the need for an emergency laparotomy. Ultrasound or CT has replaced diagnostic peritoneal lavage

  ❑ An abbreviated ultrasound examination aimed at assessing whether intra-abdominal free fluid is increasing, rather than defining the exact site of injury, is an excellent protocol when triaging patients who might require urgent surgery. This approach is known as a FAST study (= *focussed assessment for the sonographic examination of the trauma patient*). Carrying out a FAST study has been shown to be within the capabilities of residents working in the Emergency Department[12–16]

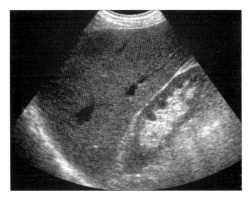

  ❑ Compressive or penetrating injuries can damage the solid organs. CT is the preferred imaging investigation for evaluating the liver, spleen and other structures in the haemodynamically stable patient

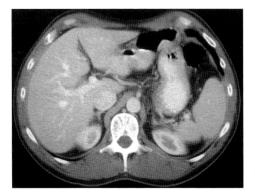

■ The severely injured **haemodynamically unstable patient** requires immediate surgery, not imaging

## KEY POINTS

### ACUTE ABDOMINAL PAIN

■ Perforation – 1.0 ml of free air can be demonstrated

■ Mechanical obstruction or paralytic ileus? Clinical correlation and analysis of the gas pattern will usually indicate whether a mechanical obstruction or a paralytic ileus is present

■ Renal colic – a limited IVU (usually only one film) is highly accurate in confirming or excluding the diagnosis. CT is an accurate alternative.

### ABDOMINAL TRAUMA

■ Delay is dangerous. Plain abdominal radiography not useful and not indicated

■ Ultrasound and/or CT are really useful in the haemodynamically stable patient.

## THE SUBTLE SIGN NOT TO MISS

| Presentation | Finding | Virtually pathognomonic of |
|---|---|---|
| Severe colicky abdominal pain | Erect AXR ... tiny pockets of gas give a 'string of beads' appearance/configuration | Mechanical obstruction to the small bowel |

## REFERENCES

1. Baker SR. Plain films and cross-sectional imaging for acute abdominal pain: unresolved issues. Semin Ultrasound CT MRI 1999; 20: 142–147.
2. de Lacey GJ, Wignall BK, Bradbrooke S et al. Rationalising abdominal radiography in the Accident and Emergency Department. Clin Radiol 1980; 31: 453–455.
3. Jelinek GA, Banham NDG. Reducing the use of plain abdominal radiographs in an emergency department. Arch Emerg Med 1990; 7: 241–245.
4. Miller RE, Nelson SW. The roentgenologic demonstration of tiny amounts of free intraperitoneal gas: experimental and clinical studies. Am J Roentgenol 1971; 112: 574–585.
5. Field S, Guy P, Upsdell SM, Scourfield AE. The erect abdominal radiograph in the acute abdomen: should its routine use be abandoned? Br Med J 1985; 290: 1934–1936.
6. Gammill SL, Nice CM. Air fluid levels: their occurrence in normal patients and their role in the analysis of ileus. Surgery 1972; 71: 771–780.
7. Maglinte DDT, Balthazar EJ, Kelvin FM, Megibow AJ. The role of radiology in the diagnosis of small bowel obstruction. AJR 1997; 168: 1171–1180.
8. Maglinte DDT, Kelvin FM, Rowe MG et al. Small bowel obstruction: optimizing radiologic investigation and non-surgical management. Radiology 2001; 218: 39–46.
9. Levine JA, Neitlich J, Verga M et al. Ureteral calculi in patients with flank pain: correlation of plain radiography with unenhanced helical CT. Radiology 1999; 204: 27–31.
10. Platt JF, Rubin JM, Ellus JH. Acute renal obstruction: evaluation with intrarenal duplex Doppler and conventional ultrasound. Radiology 1993; 186: 685–688.
11. Enderson BL, Maull KI. Missed injuries. The trauma surgeon's nemesis. Surg Clin North Am 1991; 71: 399–418.
12. Lingawi SS, Buckley AR. Focused abdominal US in patients with trauma. Radiology 2000; 217: 426–429.
13. McKenney KL. Ultrasound of blunt abdominal trauma. Radiol Clin North Am 1999; 37: 879–893.
14. Brown MA, Casola G, Sirlin CB et al. Blunt abdominal trauma: screening US in 2,693 patients. Radiology 2001; 218: 352–358.
15. Weisthaupt D, Grozaj AM, Willmann JK et al. Traumatic injuries: imaging of abdominal and pelvic injuries. Eur Radiol 2002; 12: 1295–1311.
16. Ingeman JE, Plewa MC, Okasinski RE et al. Emergency physician use of ultrasonography in blunt abdominal trauma. Acad Emerg Med 1996; 10: 931–937.

# 17 PENETRATING FOREIGN BODIES

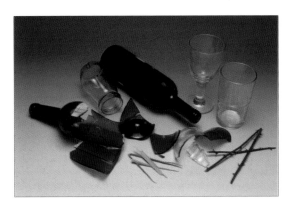

GLASS

## DETECTION

- All glass is radio-opaque. The visibility of glass is not dependent on its lead content[1,2]

- Radiographic technique is important. A soft tissue exposure is essential

- Overlying bone will hide glass fragments. The site of injury needs to be projected away from bone. Two or more projections are essential (Figs 17.1, 17.2)

- A magnifying glass or 'zooming' a digital image is often necessary. Very small fragments are easily overlooked.

## REMOVAL

Plain films will be of limited assistance when the surgeon attempts to remove a fragment situated deep in the tissues. Ultrasound is much more helpful, and can assist with the removal of any foreign body by providing precise localisation. Also it will help to minimise surgical searching and consequent soft tissue damage.

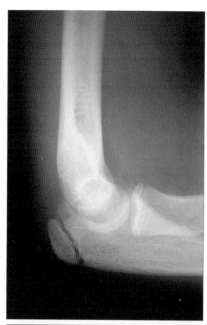

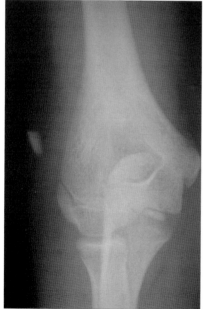

**Figure 17.1** *A dense glass fragment is hidden by bone on the lateral radiograph. It is only detected when the site of injury is projected clear of the bone on the AP view.*

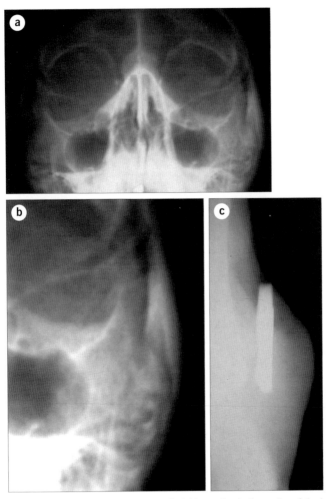

**Figure 17.2** *Assault with a bottle – facial laceration in the region of the left zygoma. On the occipitomental (OM) view **(a, b)** bone partially obscures a large fragment of glass. An oblique radiograph **(c)** projects the soft tissues deep to the laceration off the bone and the large glass fragment is clearly seen.*

**Pitfall:** A patient falls from a height through a glass roof and sustains a laceration to the upper thigh. With this history it would be insufficient to obtain films solely of the area immediately adjacent to the wound. The deep soft tissues, clear of bone, must be included. Whenever there is a history of a significant penetrative force then the area to be radiographed must take this into account.

## WOOD OR PLASTIC

### DETECTION

■ Wood splinters are occasionally radio-opaque[3] but most are impossible to detect with plain film radiography. Occasionally, a splinter will be seen on the radiograph if the fragment has paint on its surface (Fig. 17.3)

■ Detection of a wood splinter, a thorn or a plastic fragment is best undertaken with ultrasound.[4–6]

### REMOVAL

Plain film radiography is not useful. Ultrasound can be very helpful in providing guidance during exploration.[4] In exceptionally difficult cases CT or MRI will provide excellent localisation prior to surgery.

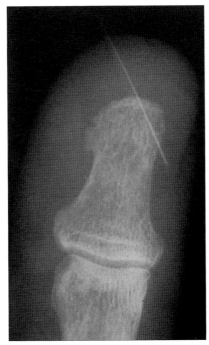

**Figure 17.3** *This splinter of wood was only visible because it had a thick coat of paint on its surface. It is usually very difficult to visualise wooden splinters or thorns on a radiograph.*

## FOREIGN BODIES IN THE ORBIT

### DETECTION

Most foreign bodies should be detected with slit lamp ophthalmoscopy.
Plain radiography, ultrasound or CT will be of assistance in selected cases.

### Metal or glass fragments

- Plain film radiography is recommended – two frontal projections (upward and then downward gaze). The movement of a fragment on upward and downward gaze will indicate whether it is situated within or outside the globe (Fig. 17.4)

- CT is available (Fig. 17.5) should there be any lack of certainty as to position after the plain films have been scrutinised.

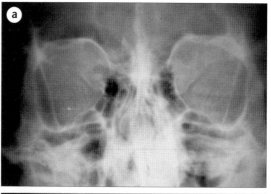

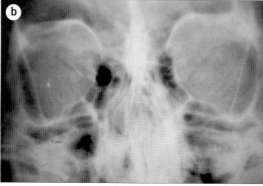

**Figure 17.4** *A metallic foreign body within the right orbit. Radiographs obtained with the patient looking down **(a)** and looking up **(b)**. The position of the fragment changes. This confirms that it lies within the globe.*

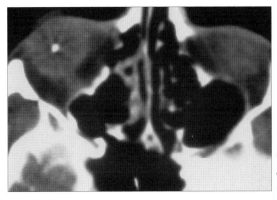

**Figure 17.5** *CT examination demonstrates the precise position of a metallic foreign body within the right orbit.*

## Wood or plastic fragments

- Ultrasound is recommended. The accuracy of detection is dependent on an experienced operator and the quality of the equipment[7]

- CT is an alternative to ultrasound. CT is sensitive, shows the retrobulbar space better than ultrasound, and is less operator-dependent.[8]

## REMOVAL

Ultrasound or CT can provide accurate localisation prior to exploration.[7,8]

## KEY POINTS – 1

### FOREIGN BODY IN THE SOFT TISSUES

- Detection
  - Metal or glass – plain film radiography is excellent
  - Thorns or splinters – ultrasound is the examination of choice
- Removal – precise localisation
  - Ultrasound in most instances
  - CT or MRI for a few exceptionally difficult cases
  - MRI contraindicated for ferromagnetic foreign bodies.

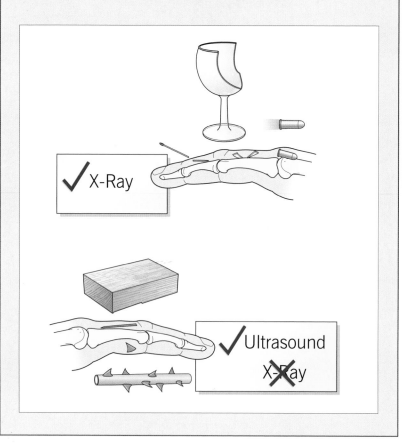

## KEY POINTS – 2

## FOREIGN BODY IN THE ORBIT

■ Clinical examination with slit lamp ophthalmoscopy will detect most foreign bodies

■ Imaging is secondary to ophthalmoscopy

■ Imaging (when needed)

❏ Metal fragments – plain film radiography

❏ Wood or plastic – ultrasound or CT; occasionally MRI.

## REFERENCES

1. Tandberg D. Glass in the hand and foot. Will an X-ray show it? JAMA 1982; 248: 1872–1874.
2. de Lacey G, Evans R, Sandin B. Penetrating injuries: how easy is it to see glass (and plastic) on radiographs? Br J Radiol 1985; 58: 27–30.
3. Roobottom CA, Weston MJ. The detection of foreign bodies in soft tissue – comparison of conventional and digital radiography. Clin Radiol 1994; 49: 330–332.
4. Gilbert FJ, Campbell RSD, Bayliss AP. The role of ultrasound in the detection of non-radiopaque foreign bodies. Clin Radiol 1990; 41: 109–112.
5. Ginsburg MJ, Ellis GL, Flom LL. Detection of soft-tissue foreign bodies by plain radiography, xerography, computed tomography, and ultrasonography. Ann Emerg Med 1990; 19: 701–703.
6. Schlesinger AE, Hernandez RJ. Diseases of the musculoskeletal system in children: imaging with CT, sonography, and MR. Am J Radiol 1992; 158: 729–741.
7. McElvanney AM, Fielder AR. Intraocular foreign body missed by radiography. Br Med J 1993; 306: 1060–1061.
8. Etherington RJ, Hourihan MD. Localisation of intraocular and intraorbital foreign bodies using computed tomography. Clin Radiol 1989; 40: 610–614.

# 18 SWALLOWED FOREIGN BODIES

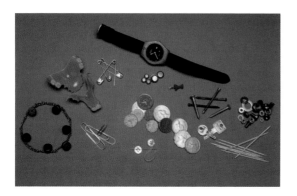

## SMALL BLUNT OBJECTS, INCLUDING COINS

### CHILDREN

■ A radiograph of the abdomen (AXR) represents unjustified radiation exposure (Fig. 18.1). It is unnecessary[1–5]

■ There is no danger to the child if the coin lies within the stomach or the intestine. (See Caution 1)

■ Occasionally, a coin may lodge in the oesophagus (Figs 18.2–18.3). Some of these patients may be asymptomatic. Erosion of the mucosa by a coin can cause an abscess or mediastinitis[2,6]

■ **Consider an alternative to radiography.** Hand-held metal detector scanning is an accurate, inexpensive, radiation-free screening tool. It can be used to examine patients suspected of ingesting coins or coin-like metallic foreign bodies[7].

### Radiography

■ A single frontal chest radiograph (CXR) to include the neck

■ No abdominal radiography.[2,4,5] If the CXR is normal, then the parents can be reassured that the coin has passed into the gut, will cause no harm and will be excreted within the next few days.

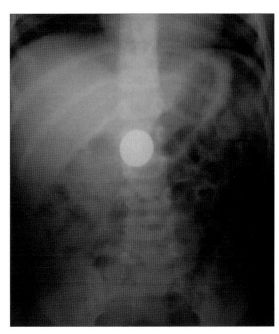

**Figure 18.1** *Swallowed coin. Abdominal radiography is not indicated and represents unjustified radiation exposure. A coin that has passed beyond the oesophagus will do no harm.*

**Caution 1** Presently, coins in the UK are inert. Elsewhere, this is not always so. Some countries have minted zinc coins with a copper coating. Gastric acid can dissolve the copper, and ingesting zinc can cause ulcers and anaemia.

In countries where coins are potentially poisonous an AXR (followed by a CXR if negative) would represent correct practice.

**Caution 2** Small bonded magnets (magnetic beads) may be harmful. Magnetic beads are present in some necklaces and bracelets worn by devotees of folk medicine. When a child plays with the necklace the string may break and small powerful magnets may enter the mouth.

A single swallowed magnet is not a problem. If several are swallowed then they can attract each other across loops of gut.[8,9] Bowel loops may be pulled together causing obstruction, perforation or a fistula.

A CXR and an AXR are indicated in children suspected of swallowing magnetic beads. If more than one bead is present, very careful monitoring is required.

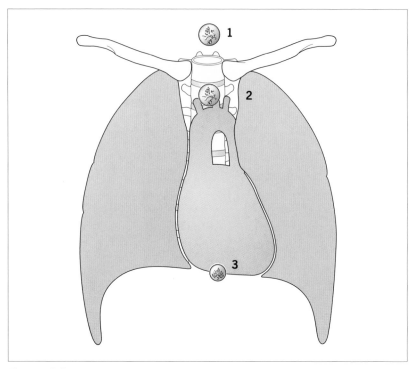

**Figure 18.2** *A coin may impact in the oesophagus. There are three sites at which hold-up most frequently occurs. 1 = cervical oesophagus; 2 = level of aortic arch; 3 = gastro-oesophageal junction.*

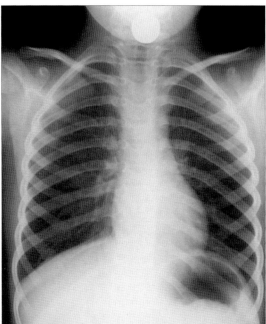

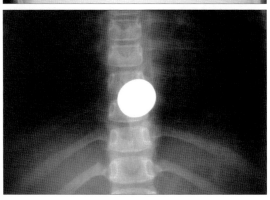

**Figure 18.3** *Swallowed coins. Chest radiography is always indicated. Two different patients. A coin can impact in the neck, at the level of the aortic arch, or at the lower end of the oesophagus. Very occasionally a coin will remain impacted and erode the mucosa. In young children the neck must always be included on the AP chest radiograph.*

## ADULTS

■ In the adult the vertebral bodies and mediastinal structures are dense. These structures are superimposed over the oesophagus on the frontal CXR. Consequently it is not always easy to detect a dense metallic object (Fig. 18.4)

■ On the lateral CXR the mid and lower oesophagus are not obscured by dense tissues. A radio-opaque foreign body will be obvious (Fig. 18.5).

### Radiography

■ Well-penetrated PA and lateral CXRs – no abdominal radiography.

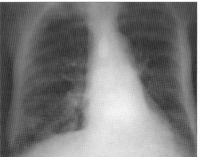

**Figure 18.4** *Adult. A swallowed coin has impacted at the level of the aortic arch. It is only just visible on this frontal chest radiograph.*

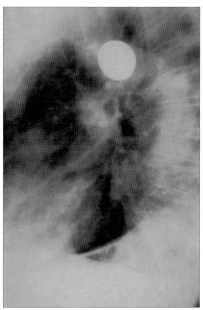

**Figure 18.5** *Lateral CXR of the same patient as in Figure 18.4. A radio-opaque foreign body that impacts in the adult oesophagus is most easily seen on the lateral view.*

## LARGE OBJECTS IN ADULTS

A large object such as a dental plate or appliance may lodge in the cervical or thoracic oesophagus (Figs 18.6, 18.7). If it remains impacted it may erode the mucosa[10,11] and cause an abscess or mediastinitis. Caution: not all dentures are radio-opaque and plain films may appear normal.

### Radiography

■ Well-penetrated PA and lateral CXRs, to include the neck

■ If these films are normal, an AXR should be obtained

■ If this film is normal, and the clinical history or symptoms remain suggestive, a barium swallow or endoscopy will be necessary.

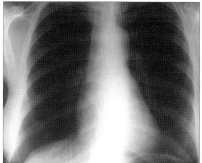

**Figure 18.6** *This patient claimed to have swallowed her dentures. No evidence of a foreign body on the PA chest radiograph. She was discharged.*

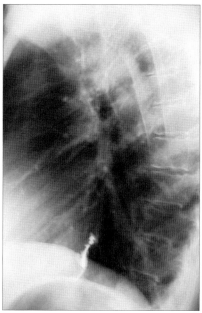

**Figure 18.7** *The patient in Figure 18.6 was recalled for a lateral CXR. The impacted denture is now obvious.*

## FISH BONES AND CHICKEN BONES

■ Bones that penetrate the gastrointestinal tract tend to lodge in the laryngopharynx or upper oesophagus[10,12]

■ Not all fish bones are calcified and the radio-opacity of the bones will vary.[13]

**Table 18.1** Radiographic density of fish bones

| Readily visible (Fig. 18.8) | More difficult to see | Not visible |
|---|---|---|
| Cod | Grey mullet | Herring |
| Haddock | Plaice | Kipper |
| Cole fish | Monkfish | Salmon |
| Lemon sole | Red snapper | Mackerel |
| Gurnard | | Trout |
| | | Pike |

### Useful anatomy

■ The soft tissue shadow between the vertebral bodies and the airway is composed of the prevertebral tissues and (below C6) the oesophagus

**Table 18.2** Normal soft tissue measurements

| Above C4 vertebra | Up to 7 mm |
|---|---|
| Below C4 vertebra | Up to 22 mm |

■ The laryngeal cartilages ossify in a variable fashion. Sometimes normal ossification (Figs 18.9–18.12) can be interpreted as a calcified foreign body. Conversely, an impacted chicken/fish bone may be incorrectly dismissed as cartilage ossification (Figs 18.12, 18.13)

■ An ossified stylohyoid ligament can mimic a bone impacted in the vallecula.

## Radiography – and what to look for

■ A soft tissue lateral radiograph of the neck[1,12]

■ Direct signs (a bone) or indirect signs (prevertebral soft tissue swelling or gas in an abscess/perforation) may be present (Fig. 18.13)

■ It is important to maintain a low threshold for proceeding to endoscopy. Apply this rule:

*If the radiograph is normal and the patient is considered well enough to be sent home, then the patient should be told to re-attend the next day if symptoms are persisting. Patients who re-attend should be seen immediately by an ear, nose and throat specialist.*

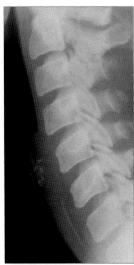 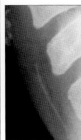

**Figure 18.8** *Impacted calcified fish bone anterior to C6 and C7 vertebrae.*

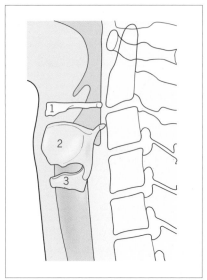

**Figure 18.9** *Normal sites of ossification/calcification*
*1 = Hyoid bone;*
*2 = thyroid cartilage;*
*3 = cricoid cartilage.*

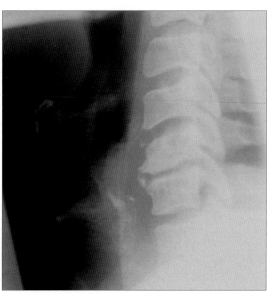

**Figure 18.10** *Pitfalls:*
*Cartilage ossification is very variable. Errors can occur through misinterpreting normal ossification or dismissing an impacted fish bone or chicken bone as normal ossification. Also, a cervical spine osteophyte can sometimes mimic an impacted foreign body. Numerous calcifications/ossifications are present in the neck of this middle aged patient.*

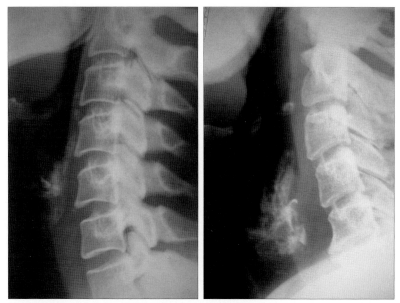

**Figure 18.11** *Normal soft tissues. Two different patients. The extent of normal ossification in the laryngeal cartilages is very variable.*

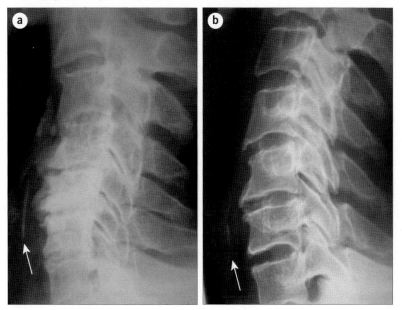

**Figure 18.12** *Pitfall: the patient (a) has swallowed a chicken bone (arrow). The patient (b) shows a somewhat similar appearance (arrow) – but this is ossification in the cricoid cartilage. An experienced observer should be consulted whenever there is any doubt.*

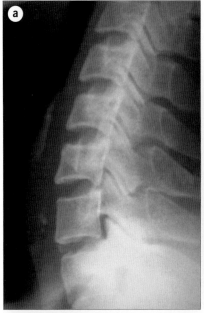

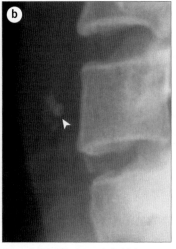

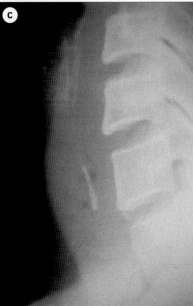

**Figure 18.13** *Impacted chicken bone. On presentation (a, b) the bone (arrowhead) lay in a horizontal position and was not recognised. Several days later (c) the bone is easy to identify as it now lies vertically. Note the soft-tissue swelling and faint bubbles of gas, indicating an abscess around a perforation. (With permission from Remedios et al[1].)*

## INANIMATE OBJECTS: SHARP OR POTENTIALLY POISONOUS

■ A **sharp or pointed object** may penetrate the bowel. Its presence needs to be confirmed or excluded (Figs 18.14, 18.15)

■ **Poisonous objects:** Very occasionally the contents of a swallowed disc/button battery may leak out.[1,14–16] Most modern disc batteries contain sodium or potassium hydroxide, which is corrosive. Some contain mercury, which is poisonous. Soft tissue damage may occasionally result from an electrical current produced by a battery and this can cause tissue necrosis.[14,15]

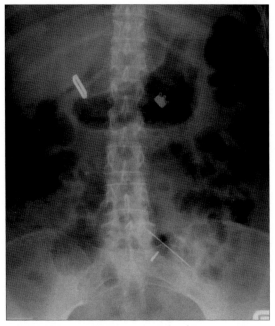

**Figure 18.14** *An AXR must be obtained whenever a sharp metallic object might have been swallowed. (This was a case of habitual foreign body ingestion. The needle places the patient at risk of a perforation.)*

## Radiography

■ An abdominal radiograph (Fig. 18.15)

  ❑ If a swallowed battery is demonstrated on the AXR, radiography should be repeated every 24 hours. If there is any sign of delay or disintegration, then endoscopic or surgical removal needs urgent consideration

  ❑ If a sharp object (e.g. needle, razor blade) is identified, management will usually be expectant. The purpose of radiography is to exclude or confirm the presence of a potentially dangerous object

■ If the expected foreign body is not seen on the AXR, then a frontal and (in the adult) a lateral CXR should be obtained

■ In some patients the AXR and CXRs will be negative and yet clinical concern remains high. Early recourse to CT is advisable

■ If an ingested sharp or pointed foreign body is non-metallic (e.g. a toothpick), plain film radiography will not identify it. Clinical management is invariably expectant.[17] If symptoms cause concern, then a CT examination is indicated.

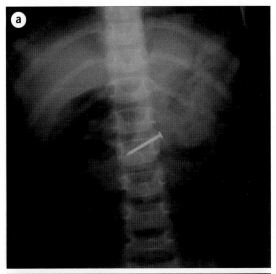

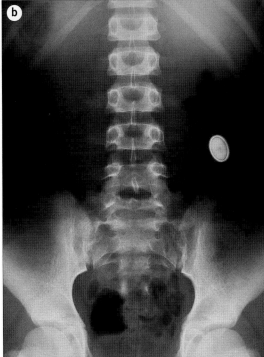

**Figure 18.15** *Two different patients. (a) The nail places the patient at a slight risk of perforation. (b) The button battery contains toxic material; very occasionally the contents of a battery can leak out through a break in the solder. Button batteries vary in size – this is the larger version.*

## KEY POINTS

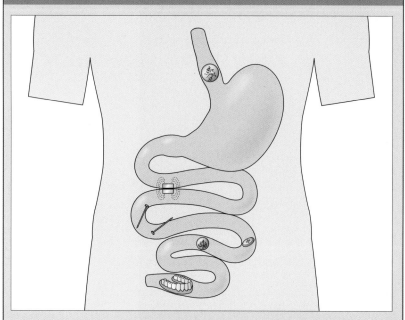

- Coins
  - AXR not indicated (but check if the local national coins are inert)
  - Children: single well-penetrated frontal CXR to include the neck
  - Adults: frontal and lateral CXRs to include the neck
  - Consider using a hand-held metal detector to detect coins.
- Sharp or potentially poisonous objects
  - AXR – if this is normal, obtain a frontal CXR in children, a frontal and a lateral CXR in adults
- Large objects in adults
  - Frontal and lateral CXRs – if normal, obtain an AXR
  - If the CXR and AXR are normal, consider a barium swallow or endoscopy
- Fish and chicken bones
  - Lateral neck radiograph
  - If the radiograph is normal and the patient is fit for discharge, explicit instructions need to be given: *'If symptoms are still present after 24 hours, please return and you will be seen by the ear, nose and throat specialist.'*

## REFERENCES

1. Remedios D, Charlesworth C, deLacey G. Imaging of foreign bodies. Imaging 1993; 5: 171–179.
2. Cooke MW, Glucksman EE. Swallowed coins. Br Med J 1991; 302: 1607.
3. Park C. Seeing is believing. Br Med J 1993; 307: 1010.
4. Stringer MD, Capps SNJ. Rationalising the management of swallowed coins in children. Br Med J 1991; 302: 1321–1322.
5. Swallowed coins. Editorial. Lancet 1989; 2: 659–660.
6. Nahman B, Meubler C. Asymptomatic oesophageal perforation by a coin in a child. Ann Emerg Med 1984; 13: 627–629.
7. Seikel K, Primm PA, Elizondo BJ et al. Hand-held metal detector localisation of ingested metallic foreign bodies; accurate in any hands? Arch Pediatr Adolesc Med 1999; 153: 853–857.
8. Lee SK, Beck NS, Kim HH. Mischievous magnets: unexpected health hazard in children. J Paediatr Surg 1996; 31: 1694–1695.
9. McCormick SR, Brennan PO, Yassa JG. Magnets and children – an attractive combination. Br Med J 2000; 321: 514.
10. Remsen K, Biller HF, Lawson W, Som L. Unusual presentations of penetrating foreign bodies of the upper aerodigestive tract. Ann Otol Rhinol Laryngol Suppl 1983; 105: 32–44.
11. Nandi P, Ong GB. Foreign body in the oesophagus: review of 2394 cases. Br J Surg 1978; 65: 5–9.
12. Herdman RCD, Saeed SR, Hinton EA. The lateral soft tissue X-ray in accident and emergency medicine. Arch Emerg Med 1991; 8: 149–156.
13. Ell SR, Sprigg A. The radio-opacity of fishbones – species variation. Clin Radiol 1991; 44: 104–107.
14. Litovitz T, Schmitz BF. Ingestion of cylindrical and button batteries: an analysis of 2382 cases. Pediatrics 1992; 89: 747–757.
15. McCombe A, Ramadan M. Severe tissue destruction in the ear caused by alkaline button batteries. Postgrad Med 1990; 66: 52–53.
16. Votteler T, Nash J, Rutledge J. The hazards of alkaline disk batteries in children. JAMA 1983; 249: 2504–2506.
17. Velitchkov NG, Grigorov GI, Losanoff JE, Kjossev KT. Ingested foreign bodies of the gastrointestinal tract: retrospective analysis of 542 cases. World J Surg 1996; 20: 1001–1005.

# 19 PARTICULAR PAEDIATRIC POINTS

Several important topics are addressed elsewhere:

|  | Chapter | Page |
|---|---|---|
| Shoulder | 4 | 68 |
| Elbow | 5 | 90 |
| Pelvis | 10 | 180 |
| Foot | 13 | 216 |
| Swallowed foreign bodies | 18 | 290 |
| Skull – normal and accessory sutures | 2 | 16 |

## LONG BONES – GENERAL

### GROWTH PLATE INJURIES: SALTER–HARRIS FRACTURES

■ The growth plate is a vulnerable structure in the paediatric skeleton. The joint capsule, the surrounding ligaments and the muscle tendons are all much stronger than the cartilaginous growth plate. A shearing or avulsion force at a joint is likely to result in an injury at the weakest point – i.e. a fracture through the growth plate

■ Failure to recognise an epiphyseal abnormality may result in suboptimal treatment. There is a risk of premature fusion of the growth plate, resulting in limb shortening. If only part of the plate is injured, unequal growth may lead to deformity and disability

■ Growth plate injuries have been classified by Salter and Harris (Fig. 19.1). This classification links the radiographic appearance to the clinical importance of the fracture: a Salter–Harris type 1 injury has a good prognosis whereas type 5 has a poor prognosis (Table 19.1).

**Type 1** is a fracture restricted to the growth plate (Fig. 19.2). Often, there is no displacement of the epiphysis and consequently it is impossible to detect the injury on the radiograph. Prognosis is very good.
**Types 2–4** represent various patterns of fracture involving the growth plate and the adjacent metaphysis and/or epiphysis (Figs 19.3–19.5). Type 4 runs the risk of premature fusion of part of the growth plate.

**Type 5** is an impaction fracture of the entire growth plate. There is little or no malalignment and it can be extremely difficult to make the diagnosis on the initial radiographs. This is the most significant of all the Salter–Harris injuries. The plate may fuse prematurely with consequent limb shortening. Diagnosis and subsequent management depends on a high degree of suspicion following clinical examination.

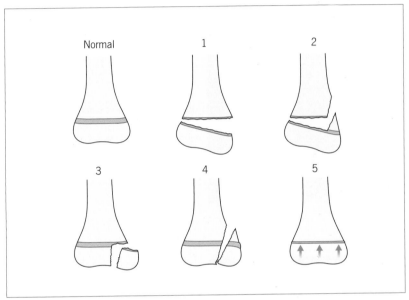

**Figure 19.1** *Epiphyseal fractures. The Salter–Harris classification.*

**Table 19.1** Salter–Harris fractures

| Type | Relative frequency[1] | Prognosis for normal growth[2] | |
|------|----------------------|-------------------|-----------|
| | | **Upper limb** | **Lower limb** |
| 1 | 8% | Satisfactory | The likelihood of a growth complication is higher for all types of Salter–Harris injury – as compared with the upper limb |
| 2 | 73% | Satisfactory | |
| 3 | 6% | Satisfactory | |
| 4 | 12% | Guarded | |
| 5 | 1% | Poor | |

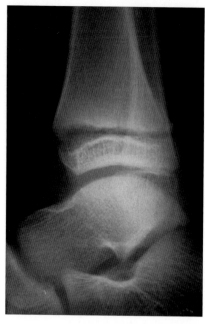

**Figure 19.2** *Salter–Harris type 1 injury. Widening of the tibial growth plate anteriorly. The normal growth plate should show an even space between the epiphysis and the metaphysis.*

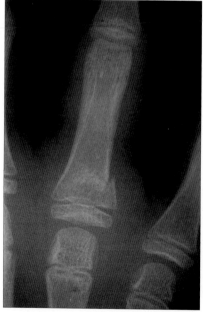

**Figure 19.3** *Salter–Harris type 2 injury. A fracture through the metaphysis of the proximal phalanx extending into the epiphyseal plate.*

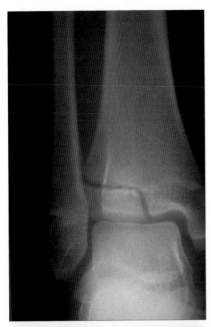

**Figure 19.4** *Salter–Harris type 3 injury. A fracture through the distal tibial epiphysis extending into the epiphyseal plate. The lateral aspect of the growth plate is widened.*

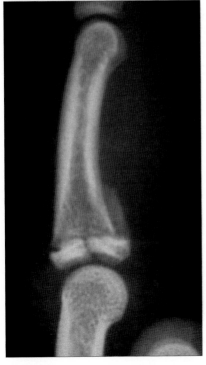

**Figure 19.5** *Salter–Harris type 4 injury. The fracture involves the epiphyseal plate, the epiphysis and the metaphysis.*

## GREENSTICK, TORUS AND PLASTIC BOWING FRACTURES

These only occur in children. They differ from fractures in adults because the child's skeleton is elastic. When a child's long bone is subjected to a longitudinal compression force (e.g. fall on an outstretched hand) this can result in three different types of injury:

- **Greenstick fracture**. Results from an angulation force. There is a break in the cortex on one side of the bone. The opposite cortex remains intact (Figs 19.6, 19.7). This occurs because a child's periosteum is both elastic and very thick. There is usually angulation at the fracture site, although this can be subtle

- **Torus fracture**. Results from a longitudinal compression force with little or no angulation. There are microfractures of the trabeculae at the injured site. Instead of a break in the cortex there is just a slight buckling (Figs 19.7, 19.8). The commonest sites are the distal radius and ulna. The fracture is often subtle and appears as a ripple, a wave or a slight bump in the cortex

- **Plastic bowing fracture**. A bone may simply bend or bow with no obvious break in the cortex. The mechanism is as follows: longitudinal compression causes the bone to bend and the concave surface develops a series of microfractures. The compression force is insufficient to cause a greenstick or transverse fracture (Fig. 19.9)

  - ❏ Plastic bowing fractures usually involve the radius or ulna. Sometimes they can be difficult to diagnose with certainty because differences in radiographic positioning of the normal forearm bones can mimic a slightly bent bone

  - ❏ Frequently a plastic bowing fracture is only recognised in retrospect when subsequent films show periosteal new bone extending along the cortex.

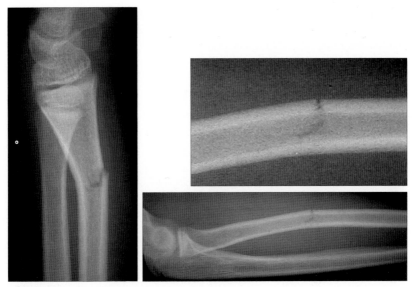

**Figure 19.6** *Greenstick fractures. Slight angulation is present in both cases.*

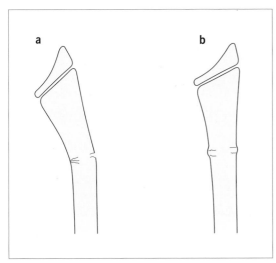

**Figure 19.7** *(a) Greenstick fracture: cortical break with angulation. (b) Torus fracture – cortical buckling but no angulation.*

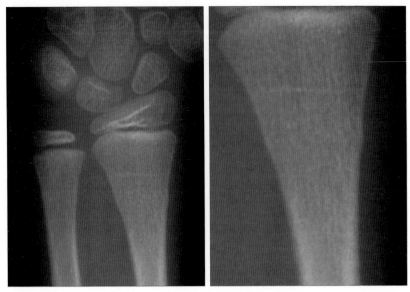

**Figure 19.8** *Torus fracture – buckling of the radial cortex; no angulation.*

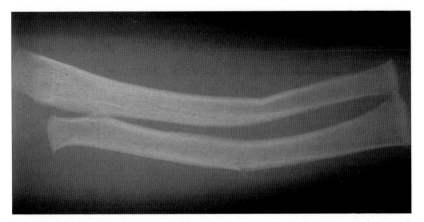

**Figure 19.9** *Plastic bowing fracture of the ulna. There is an associated greenstick fracture of the radius.*

## ELBOW

### Pulled (nursemaid's) elbow
Described on page 94 in Chapter 5.

■ A sudden pull on the hand with the elbow extended may cause the radial head to sublux. The clinical diagnosis is usually obvious, and reduction is achieved simply by supinating the forearm. A successful reduction is accompanied by immediate relief of symptoms

■ When the clinical features are typical, radiography is not indicated.

### Supracondylar fracture
Described on page 98 in Chapter 5.

### Injuries involving the secondary ossification centres
Described on page 99 in Chapter 5.

## TODDLER'S FRACTURES

■ The most common toddler's fracture involves the shaft of the tibia. Usually it occurs in a child aged 9 months to 3 years. The child falls with one leg fixed and a twisting injury occurs resulting in a spiral fracture of the tibia (Fig. 19.10). Invariably, the fracture is undisplaced and is frequently difficult to visualise on the initial radiographs. Sometimes it will only be demonstrated on an additional oblique projection, or on a radionuclide study. If a repeat radiograph is obtained 10–14 days after the injury periosteal new bone will be present (Fig. 19.11)

■ Toddler's fractures also occur in the femur, cuboid, calcaneum and distal fibula.[3–7] Different jumping or stumbling mechanisms create particular forces that affect specific bones.

**Note:** If a child refuses to weight-bear or is well but limping, then the possibility of a toddler's fracture needs to be considered. If the tibia appears normal on oblique views then there are two possible courses of action:

❑ Scintigraphy will provide an assessment of the tibia and of the other bones that are occasionally the site of a fracture. In general, the role of scintigraphy is to exclude a more serious abnormality

OR:

❑ Adopt an expectant approach. Toddler's fractures heal without any particular treatment. In a limping but otherwise well child, repeat plain film radiography 10–14 days later (Fig. 19.11) will often show evidence of the healing fracture.

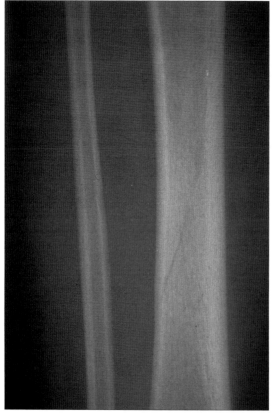

**Figure 19.10** *A toddler's fracture (spiral fracture of the middle third of the tibia).*

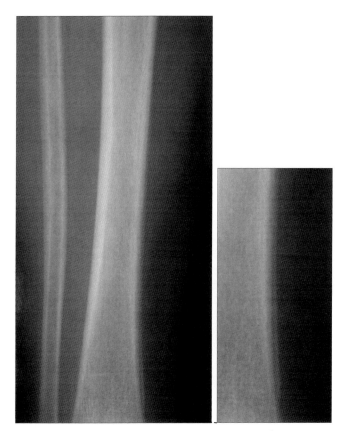

**Figure 19.11** *A well child suddenly refused to weight bear. The initial radiographs were entirely normal. Ten days later the presence of periosteal new bone confirmed the original clinical diagnosis of a toddler's fracture.*

## PAINFUL HIP IN THE ABSENCE OF TRAUMA

### Differential diagnosis

- Children with hip pain are the commonest cause of paediatric orthopaedic admissions in the UK

- The patient's age will give some idea as to the most likely cause of hip pain

  - **Irritable hips** occur in both sexes throughout childhood

  - **Perthes'** disease is more common in boys and is rare over the age of 7 years

  - **Slipped femoral capital epiphysis** (SFCE) is more common in boys. It is rare under the age of 8 years

- Infants and toddlers may be brought to the Emergency Department because they are reluctant to move a leg, but without any direct hip signs or symptoms. Most of these children are eventually diagnosed as having a transient synovitis (irritable hip), which is a self-limiting condition associated with a joint effusion. It is presumed to be of viral aetiology. Rarely, a more serious abnormality such as septic arthritis or Perthes' disease is the cause.

### Investigation of the painful hip

Practice varies between centres. The following is a formal protocol employed in children presenting to the Emergency Department with hip pain or reluctant to move a leg. In some centres, plain radiographs are only obtained if the ultrasound examination is normal.[8]

1. The patient is registered under the care of the specialist paediatric or orthopaedic team

2. On admission to the Emergency Department local anaesthetic cream is placed on the hip skin crease

3. Plain frontal and frog-leg pelvic radiographs are obtained. If:

   - Obvious bone abnormality – **stop**

   - Radiographs are normal – **proceed to**:

4. Immediate hip ultrasound for confirmation or exclusion of a joint effusion

5. In every case of effusion, synovial fluid is aspirated under ultrasound control. Immediate Gram stain is performed. If positive, antibiotic treatment is started. If negative, the child may be safely discharged home whilst awaiting the result of culture – *provided that the family is within easy reach by telephone*

6. All children are reviewed 1 week later in the paediatric or orthopaedic clinic. If symptoms persist a radionuclide study is obtained in order to exclude early Perthes' disease or other rare causes of hip pain such as osteomyelitis, bone tumour or stress fracture of the femoral neck.

Using this protocol the painful hip is transformed from the most common cause of paediatric orthopaedic hospital admission into a condition which can be managed as an outpatient.[8]

## AVULSION FRACTURES

■ Descriptions of the common apophyseal avulsion injuries are included under Pelvis (page 186), Elbow (page 102), and Midfoot and forefoot (page 231)

■ These apophyseal fractures are common in athletic children and adolescents[9,10]

   ❏ An apophysis is a secondary ossification centre that is not related to a joint surface

   ❏ Apophyses are often the sites of tendonous insertions

   ❏ Avulsion occurs as a result of a violent or repetitive muscle pull

   ❏ In effect an apophyseal fracture is a growth plate injury and is analogous to a Salter–Harris type I fracture.

## HEAD INJURY

■ See Chapter 2, pages 28–43

■ There are numerous normal appearances which may be confusing. It is often necessary to consult Keats' *Atlas*[11] or to seek the opinion of an experienced observer.

## ACCESSORY SUTURES

■ Accessory sutures (complete or incomplete) are normal in neonates and young children (Figs 19.12–19.14). Any of these sutures may be misinterpreted as a fracture, conversely a fracture may be dismissed as an accessory suture

■ In the context of non-accidental injury (NAI) an awareness of the position of these sutures is important. An extensive description of accessory sutures is provided in Chapter 2, pages 28–43.

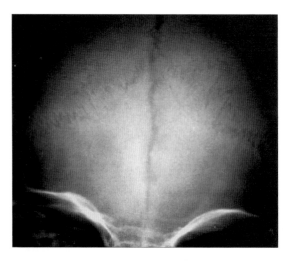

**Figure 19.12** *The metopic suture is present in this frontal bone, a normal variant.*

**Figure 19.13** *The spheno-occipital synchondrosis (arrow). A normal appearance.*

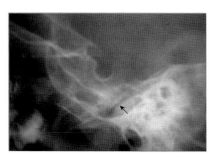

**Figure 19.14**
*An incomplete accessory parietal suture situated just above the lambdoid suture.*

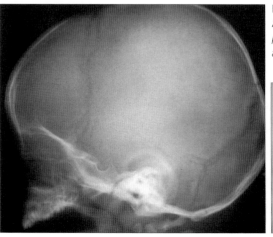

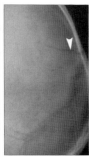

## WIDENING OF SUTURES

Following a head injury a suture may show diastasis (i.e. widening) due to either a fracture through the suture or increased pressure from an intracranial haematoma. Occasionally, sutural widening may be the only evidence of injury (Fig. 19.15).

---

**Pitfall:** The widths of the normal sutures are variable. An experienced observer will often be required to provide reassurance as to whether or not a particular appearance lies within the normal range.

---

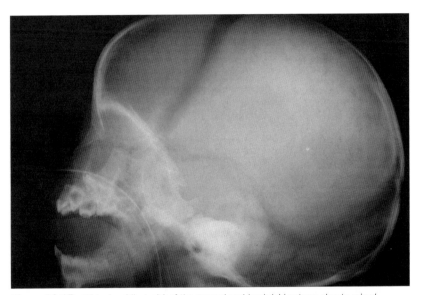

**Figure 19.15** *Widening (diastasis) of the coronal and lambdoid sutures due to raised intracranial pressure. This child had been shaken violently. A subsequent CT examination revealed extensive intracranial haemorrhage. NAI.*

## NON-ACCIDENTAL INJURY

■ The possibility of non-accidental injury (NAI) needs to be considered in all injured children presenting to the Emergency Department. No socioeconomic group or race is exempt

   ❏ 50% of cases of NAI occur before the age of 1 year

   ❏ 80% occur before the age of 2 years

■ Normal radiographs do not exclude the diagnosis. In 50% of proven cases of NAI the radiographs are normal

■ A particular area of difficulty is the skull. Fractures may be confused with normal accessory sutures and vice versa. Detailed descriptions of the normal SXR in infants are included on pages 28–43.

### Radiographic features suggestive of NAI[12–18]

■ More than one fracture (Fig. 19.16). This is particularly suspicious if the stages of evolution of the fractures appear to be different, since this indicates that the injuries have occurred at different times. For example, one fracture may show a slight periosteal reaction whereas another may demonstrate mature callus formation

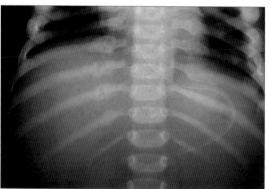
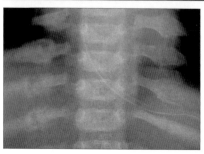

**Figure 19.16** *NAI.*
*Multiple posterior rib fractures.*

■ **Subperiosteal new bone formation**. Periosteal reactions may result from subperiosteal bleeding caused by punching, shaking or squeezing. Although periosteal reaction and callus formation can occur within a few days of trauma, neither will be present on the actual day of the injury. If new bone is present then days or weeks have elapsed since the injury (Fig. 19.17).

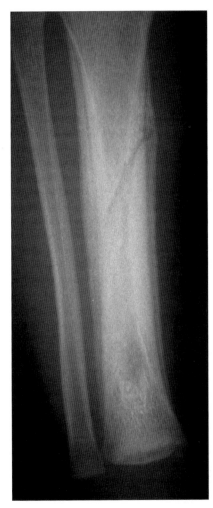

**Figure 19.17** *NAI. Periosteal new bone along the cortical margins of the tibia associated with an undisplaced fracture of the shaft.*

## Radiographic features highly suggestive/virtually pathognomonic of NAI[12,17]

- A small fracture (Fig. 19.18) at the corner of a metaphysis of a long bone. This is known as a corner fracture

- A transverse fracture of the distal metaphysis of a long bone which has been likened to a bucket handle (Figs 19.18, 19.19)

- Fractures involving the posterior aspects of the ribs close to the spine (Fig. 19.16). These occur when a child is held by the chest and shaken or squeezed

  - Rib fractures in children under the age of 2 years are usually due to NAI

  - Rib fractures often result from very violent shaking episodes – these have a recognised association with brain injury

- Fractures of the pelvis, sternum, and the vertebral transverse processes. These are rarely caused by an accidental injury

- Skull fractures that are wide, complex and involving both sides of the skull, or involving both the occiput and the vertex.

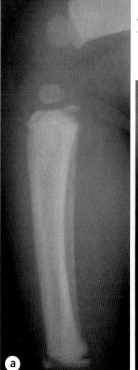
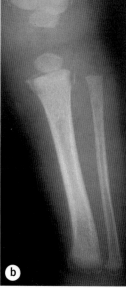
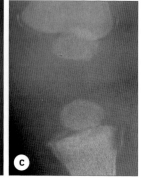

**Figure 19.18** *NAI. Corner fractures of the distal femur and proximal tibia* **(a)**. *Bucket handle fractures of the distal femur and proximal tibia* **(b, c)**.

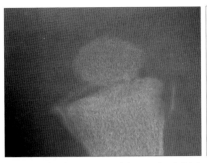 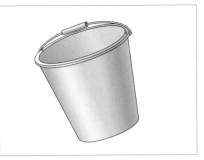

**Figure 19.19** *Fracture of the proximal tibial metaphysis. Typical appearance of a bucket handle fracture.*

## Pitfalls:

**1 :** 'The foremost pitfall in the radiologic diagnosis of abuse is suboptimal imaging, most frequently resulting from radiographic under- or overexposure and malposition.'[17]

**2 :** Normal skeletal variants may be misinterpreted as evidence of NAI. These include accessory skull sutures (pages 28–43), physiological periosteal reaction and normal metaphyseal variants.[14]

**3 :** Other pathological processes, e.g. osteogenesis imperfecta or osteomyelitis. These may simulate NAI.

## CHEST: INHALED FOREIGN BODY

The most commonly inhaled foreign body is food, frequently a peanut.[19–21] A history of choking is usually obtained. Common clinical signs include coughing, stridor, wheezing and sternal retraction. Rapid recognition and treatment are essential. This is a medical emergency.

### Radiography

■ If the child is able to cooperate then the frontal CXR should be obtained following a rapid forced expiration. Air trapping on the affected side is then more obvious (Fig. 19.20)

■ Fluoroscopy is an excellent way of noting whether there is unilateral air trapping.

### Possible findings

■ Area of collapse/consolidation

■ Unilateral hypertransradiant lung, due to air trapping. The affected lung appears blacker and larger than the opposite normal side (Fig. 19.20)

■ Normal appearances.[21] This is not necessarily reassuring. If clinical suspicion remains strong that a foreign body has been inhaled, early referral to MRI[22] or bronchoscopy is essential.

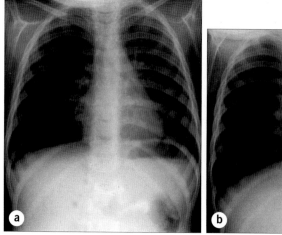
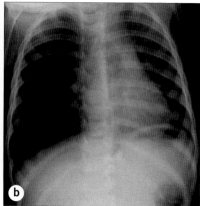

**Figure 19.20** *An inhaled peanut in the right main bronchus. Inspiration film (a); the right lung is hypertransradiant (i.e. blacker) compared with the left. Following rapid expiration (b) air trapping on the right is now obvious. Mediastinal displacement to the left is evident.*

## CHEST AND ABDOMEN: SWALLOWED FOREIGN BODIES

See Chapter 18.

## REFERENCES

1. Mizuta T, Benson WM, Foster BK et al. Statistical analysis of the incidence of physeal injuries. J Pediatr Orthop 1987; 7: 518–523.
2. Kao SCS, Smith WL. Skeletal injuries in the pediatric patient. Radiol Clin North Am 1997; 35: 727–746.
3. Swischuk LE, John SD, Tschoepe EJ. Upper tibial hyperextension fractures in infants: another occult toddler's fracture. Pediat Radiol 1999; 29: 6–9.
4. Blumber K, Patterson RJ. The toddler's cuboid fracture. Radiology 1991; 179: 93–94.
5. Laliotis N, Pennie BH, Carty H, Klenemar L. Toddler's fracture of the calcaneum. Injury 1993; 24: 169–170.
6. Donnelly LF. Toddler's fracture of the fibula. AJR 2000; 175: 922.
7. John SD, Moontry CS, Swischuk LE. Expanding the concept of the toddler's fracture. Radiographics 1997; 17: 367–376.
8. Fink M, Berman L, Edwards D, Jacobson K. Irritable hips – is there a need for hospital admission? Br J Radiol 1993; 66: 629.
9. Saunders M, Carty H. Avulsion fractures of the pelvis in children: a report of 32 fractures and their outcome. Skeletal Radiol 1994; 23: 85–90.
10. El-Khoury GY, Daniel WW, Kathol MH. Acute and chronic avulsive injuries. Radiol Clin North Am 1997; 35: 747–751.
11. Keats TE. Atlas of normal roentgen variants that may simulate disease, 7th ed. Chicago, IL: Year Book, 2001.
12. Carty H, Pierce A. Non-accidental injury: a retrospective analysis of a large cohort. Eur Radiol 2002; 12: 2919–2925.
13. Kleinman PK. Diagnostic imaging in infant abuse. AJR 1990; 155: 703–712.
14. Kleinman PK, Belanger PL, Karellas A, Spevak MR. Normal metaphyseal radiologic variants not to be confused with findings of infant abuse. AJR 1991; 156: 781–783.
15. Merten DF, Radkowski MA, Leonidas JC. The abused child: a radiological reappraisal. Radiology 1983; 146: 377–381.
16. Merten DF, Osbourne DRS. Craniocerebral trauma in the child abuse syndrome: radiological observations. Paediatr Radiol 1984; 14: 272–277.
17. Merten DF, Carpenter BL. Radiologic imaging of inflicted injury in the child abuse syndrome. Pediatr Clin North Am 1990; 37: 815–837.
18. Mogbo KI, Slovis TL, Canady AI et al. Appropriate imaging in children with skull fractures and suspicion of abuse. Radiology 1998; 208: 521–524.
19. Rothman BF, Boeckman CR. Foreign bodies in the larynx and tracheo-bronchial tree in children. Ann Otol 1980; 89: 434–436.
20. Baharloo F, Veyckemans F, Francis C et al. Tracheobronchial foreign bodies: presentation and management in children and adults. Chest 1999; 115: 1357–1362.
21. Svedstrom E, Puhakka H, Kero P. How accurate is chest radiography in the diagnosis of tracheobronchial foreign bodies in children? Pediatr Radiol 1989; 19: 520–522.
22. Imaizumi H, Kaneko M, Nara S et al. Definitive diagnosis and location of peanuts in the airways using magnetic resonance imaging techniques. Ann Emerg Med 1994; 23: 1379–1382.

Synonyms are marked aka.
UK terms are marked[1], USA terms are marked[2].

**Accessory ossicle**  Normal small bone which is present in many, but not all, individuals. These ossicles are particularly common in the foot. May be confused with a fracture fragment. The usual distinguishing features are that an ossicle has well-defined and corticated margins.

**Accessory ossification centre**  A secondary centre of ossification which is a normal variant. For example, the patella may have two or three accessory ossification centres. Sometimes these small centres never fuse to the main bone. They may be mistaken for fracture fragments.

**Accessory suture**  A suture is a joint between the bones of the skull vault. An accessory suture is one that is not usually present in the adult skull. Accessory sutures are common in neonates and infants. They disappear (i.e. fusion occurs) at variable intervals during childhood. Sometimes an accessory suture persists into adulthood. Some accessory sutures are referred to as fissures.

**Accident and Emergency Department**  See: Emergency Department.

**Adynamic ileus[2]**  aka Paralytic ileus.[1]

**AP**  Antero-posterior. Indicates the direction of the x-ray beam as it passes through the patient.

**Apophysis**  A secondary centre of ossification which affects the contour or size of a bone but does not add to its length. Muscles and tendons frequently arise from, or insert into, an apophysis.

**Atelectasis**  aka Collapse (pulmonary).

**Avulsion fracture**  A bone fragment or an apophysis that has been pulled away from the parent bone. Usually occurs at the site of insertion of a tendon or ligament. Results from excessive muscle contraction, an abnormal degree of forced movement at a joint, or chronic repetitive stress.

**Axial radiograph**  aka axial projection or axial view. The x-ray beam is directed along a plane parallel to the long axis of the body. Examples: axial view of the shoulder; axial view of the calcaneum.

**AXR[1]**  Aka KUB[2]. An abdominal radiograph.

**Bankart lesion**  A fracture of the anterior glenoid labrum involving the bone or cartilage, or both together. A potential complication of an anterior dislocation of the glenohumeral joint.

**Barton fracture**  aka Barton's fracture. A shear type fracture involving the cortex of the distal radius and its articular surface. It is unstable. The intra-articular fracture involves the dorsal margin of the radius; the carpus (when there is displacement) follows the distal fragment posteriorly.

A reverse Barton fracture is one involving the anterior cortex of the radius, including the articular surface, with the volar (anterior) fragment maintaining its relationship with the carpus. To reduce semantic misunderstandings a reverse Barton fracture is more helpfully termed a volar Barton fracture.

*Note:* Some medical texts provide confusing and erroneous descriptions. Sometimes a reverse (or volar) Barton fracture is incorrectly called a Barton fracture; sometimes a simple longitudinal intra-articular fracture (not involving the anterior or posterior cortex of the radius) is given the generic title of a Barton fracture.

**Basal joint of the thumb**  The carpometacarpal joint (i.e. the trapezium-metacarpal joint).

**Baseball finger[2]**  See: Mallet finger.[1]

**Battered baby syndrome**  See: Non-accidental injury (NAI).

**Bennett's fracture**  aka Bennett's fracture dislocation. An intra-articular fracture involving the base of the first metacarpal. Invariably associated with dislocation at the first carpo-metacarpal joint.

**Bowing fracture**  See: Plastic bowing fracture.

**Boxer's fracture**  Involving the neck of the second and / or third metacarpal. The trained boxer maintains his / her wrist in the neutral position in order to deliver the maximum impact. Contrast this with a Fighter's or Scrapper's fracture in which the untrained individual usually strikes with the wrist in the flexed position and sustains a fracture of the fourth and / or fifth metacarpal.

**Bucket handle fracture**  In children only. A metaphyseal fracture line which lies parallel to the growth plate of a long bone. It may not extend across the whole width of the bone. A shearing injury. In an infant this metaphyseal fracture is highly suggestive of a non-accidental injury (NAI). See Corner fracture.

**Buddy strapping**  See: Garter strapping.

**Bumper fracture**  See: Fender fracture.

**Button battery**  aka Disc battery. For example, in watches and electronic calculators.

**Calcaneum**  aka Calcaneus.

**Capitellum**  aka Capitulum.

**Carpal navicular[2]**  aka Scaphoid bone[1]

**Comminuted fracture**  Fragmentation of a bone into three or more parts.

**Consolidation**   Refers to the replacement of alveolar air by fluid. On a chest radiograph the affected area of lung appears white or dense. This density (i.e. consolidation) may be due to replacement of air by pus (pneumonia), by blood (pulmonary haemorrhage), or by oedema fluid. Note: the term consolidation is often used (incorrectly) as a synonym for pneumonia.

**Corner fracture**   See Bucket handle fracture. A metaphyseal fracture occurring as a result of a non-accidental injury. Sometimes the whole bucket handle configuration is not apparent but the thicker peripheral rim of the detached fragment is seen as a small triangle of bone – a corner fracture.

**CSF**   Cerebro-spinal fluid.

**CTR**   Cardio-thoracic ratio. A measurement which indicates whether the heart is likely to be enlarged or not enlarged.

**CXR**   Chest radiograph.

**Decubitus position**   The patient is reclining. In a radiographic context it is used to denote that the patient is lying on his or her side. The term implies that a horizontal beam radiograph has been obtained. This technique can be used to demonstrate free intra-abdominal air or to confirm the presence of fluid in the pleural space.

**Diaphysis**   The shaft of a long bone. It merges with the metaphysis at either end. See: Epiphysis.

**Diastasis**   Separation of normally adjacent bones with or without an associated fracture, or a separation at a site of fibro-cartilaginous union. Examples: of the tibia and fibula at the ankle mortice; at a sacroiliac joint; of a skull suture.

**Dome of the diaphragm**   aka Hemidiaphragm. The term diaphragms is sometimes used – an incorrect use of language. There is only one diaphragm separating the thorax from the abdomen. It has a right dome and a left dome.

**Dorsal**   Relating to the posterior (extensor) aspect of the body or of a body part (e.g. a limb). See: Ventral.

**Dynamic ileus**[2]   aka Mechanical obstruction.[1]

**Emergency Department**[1]   Commonly abbreviated to ED. aka Accident Department[1]; Accident and Emergency Department[1]; Casualty[1]; Emergency Room[2] (ER).

**Emergency Room**[2]   Commonly abbreviated to ER. aka Accident Department[1]; Accident and Emergency Department[1] (A and E); Casualty[1]; Emergency Department[1] (ED).

**Emperor's New Clothes**   The authors' view of vessel changes detectable on an erect chest radiograph when the pulmonary venous pressure is raised (i.e. upper lobe blood diversion). In routine practice this finding is rarely seen and is frequently equivocal. The authors (of this book) take the view that an inappropriate emphasis has been placed on this occasional, unreliable, and (in clinical practice) often disputable appearance.

**ENT surgery**[1] Ear, nose and throat surgery.[1]

**Epidural** aka Extradural.

**Epiphyseal fusion** aka Epiphyseal closure. The epiphysis when fully ossified merges with the metaphysis of the long bone. The age at which epiphyseal ossification commences and fusion (with the metaphysis) occurs varies from bone to bone. At most sites there is a slight variation in the age at which fusion occurs in males and females.

**Epiphysis** The epiphysis forms the bone-end. It enlarges by growth of cartilage within the secondary centre adjacent to the growth plate. Gradually the epiphysis ossifies. Eventually when the growth plate disappears the epiphysis fuses to the metaphysis. See: Epiphyseal fusion; Metaphysis.

**Fabella** aka Fabellum.

**Fatigue fracture** aka March fracture, Stress fracture. See: Stress fracture.

**FBI** Fat–blood interface in the suprapatellar bursa following trauma. aka lipohaemarthrosis; fat–fluid level (FFL).

**Fender fracture** aka Car bumper fracture, Bumper fracture. A fracture of a tibial plateau. Conventionally, it usually refers to a fracture of the lateral plateau.

**FFL** See: FBI.

**Fighter's fracture** aka Scrapper's fracture. A fracture through the neck of the fourth or fifth metacarpal. So named because it invariably occurs when a blow is struck by an untrained street fighter (or scrapper). The clenched fist is not kept in a neutral position. Consequently, the main force is transmitted through the lateral metacarpals. Contrast this with the trained Boxer who strikes with the clenched fist held in the neutral position and is more likely to fracture the neck of the second or third metacarpal. See: Boxer's fracture; Scrapper's fracture.

**Fluid level** Only demonstrable on a horizontal beam radiograph. May be an air–fluid or fat–fluid level (see Lipohaemarthrosis).

**Fluoroscopy**[1,2] aka Screening[1]; Fluoroscopic screening. Viewing an area of anatomy on a screen or on a monitor utilising a machine which provides a real time x-ray image. Can (for example) be used to detect air trapping in a child who may have aspirated a foreign body. Also used to assist in the manipulation of fractures.

**Galeazzi fracture-dislocation** aka Galeazzi fracture. A fracture of the shaft of the radius associated with dislocation at the distal radio-ulnar joint.

**Gamekeeper's thumb** aka Skier's thumb. Strictly speaking these are not synonymous eponyms. A Gamekeeper's thumb results from stretching of the ulnar collateral ligament of the first metacarpo-phalangeal joint (consequent on wringing rabbit necks); a Skier's thumb represents a rupture of the ligament.

**Garter strapping** aka Buddy strapping. A method of immobilising some phalangeal fractures. The injured digit is strapped to an adjacent uninjured digit.

**Greenstick fracture** A fracture of a long bone in a child. There is a break of one cortex only. Usually accompanied by some angulation at the fracture site.

**Growth plate** aka Cartilaginous growth plate, Epiphyseal plate, Epiphyseal disc. The layer of cartilage between the metaphysis and epiphysis of an unfused long bone. Sometimes referred to as the Phyis – incorrectly, because there is no such anatomical term.

**GSW** Gun shot wound.

**Hemidiaphragm** aka Dome of the diaphragm. There is only one diaphragm separating the thorax from the abdomen. It has two domes.

**Hill Sach's deformity** aka Hill Sach's lesion. A compression fracture of the postero-lateral margin of the humeral head. A potential complication of anterior dislocation of the gleno-humeral joint.

**Horizontal beam radiograph** aka Cross table radiograph. Denotes the orientation of the x-ray beam relative to the floor. The beam is parallel to the floor. This technique may be used to demonstrate a fluid level (e.g. in the supra-patellar bursa of the knee, or in the sphenoid sinus of the skull), or utilised when a patient should not be moved from the supine position (e.g. lateral cervical spine radiograph following trauma).

**Incomplete suture** aka Fissure (skull). See: Accessory suture.

**Insufficiency fracture** A fracture occurring as the result of normal stress on abnormal bone. For example – a vertebral fracture occurring without trauma / a fall in an elderly patient who has osteoporosis. These fractures are completely different in aetiology from stress (i.e. fatigue) fractures.

**Intravenous urogram (IVU)** aka Excretory urogram, Intravenous pyelogram (IVP).

**Irritable hip** aka Transient synovitis, Toxic synovitis.

**Isotope investigation** aka Nuclear medicine investigation, Radio-isotope study, Radionuclide scan, Scintiscan, Scintigraphy.

**Javelin thrower's elbow** Avulsion of the lateral (external) epicondyle of the humerus.

**Jones' fracture** A fracture of the diaphysis of the fifth metatarsal situated within 1.5cm of the tuberosity but distal to the metatarsal-cuboid joint. Occurs either as an acute injury or as a stress fracture. Not to be confused with the easily managed fracture of the tuberosity caused by an inversion injury. Recognition / distinction is important because inappropriate treatment can lead to non-union.

**Junior doctor[1]** This term includes Resident[2], Specialist registrar[1]. A doctor (e.g. physician or surgeon) training in a hospital.

**KUB[2] aka AXR[1]** An abdominal radiograph.

**Lipohaemarthrosis** Liquid fat and blood within a joint demonstrable on a horizontal beam radiograph. Most commonly seen at the knee joint when marrow fat enters the joint via an intra-articular fracture and forms a fat-fluid level (FFL). Also, sometimes seen when there has been an injury to the shoulder joint. Occasionally referred to as a fat-blood interface or FBI.

**Lisfranc joint** The tarsometatarsal joints. Usually referred to in the context of a Lisfranc fracture dislocation; the most common dislocation of the foot.

**Little leaguer's elbow**[2] Avulsion injury of the medial (internal) epicondyle of the humerus. Occurs most commonly in children – particularly those involved in throwing sports, such as baseball pitching.

**Lucent** Denotes a dark line, or dark area, on a radiograph. Commonly used as a descriptive term when indicating that a fracture is identifiable by a lucent line (or lucency).

**Lytic** The opposite of sclerotic. Denotes an area on a bone radiograph which appears darker or blacker than the adjacent normal bone. The word lytic often implies bone destruction. Sometimes used as a synonym for lucent.

**Madonna sign**[1,2] Widening of the scapho-lunate joint consequent on a ligamentous injury. Named after an iconic 21st century American singer and actress whose two upper central incisors are separated by a gap. Synonymous with the Terry Thomas sign.[1]

**Maisonneuve fracture** A fracture or ligamentous rupture at the ankle joint accompanied by a high fracture of the shaft of the fibula.

**Mallet finger**[1] aka Baseball finger.[2] A flexion deformity of a distal interphalangeal joint with or without a fracture of the dorsum at the base of the terminal phalanx. The injury is an avulsion of the extensor tendon.

**March fracture** aka Fatigue fracture, Stress fracture. It is common for the term march fracture to be used in reference (specifically) to a stress fracture of a metatarsal.

**Metaphysis** The region of bone situated between the growth plate and the shaft (diaphysis) of a long bone.

**Monteggia fracture-dislocation** aka Monteggia fracture. A fracture of the shaft of the ulna associated with dislocation of the head of the radius.

**MRI** Magnetic resonance imaging. Frequently shortened to MR.

**MVA**[2] aka Motor vehicle accident[2], Road traffic accident (RTA)[1].

**Non-accidental injury (NAI)** aka Battered baby, Battered child, Child abuse. Euphemism for a deliberate assault. Used in the context of an injury to a young child or infant.

**Nursemaid's elbow**[2] aka Pulled elbow.[1]

**Occipito-frontal radiograph of the skull (OF)** aka Caldwell projection.

**Occipito-mental radiograph of the face (OM)** aka Water's projection. A radiograph of the facial bones obtained with the axis of the x-ray beam directed between the chin and the occiput. May be followed by a number (e.g. OM 30 or OM 15) which denotes the degree of angulation of the x-ray beam.

**Odontoid peg** aka the dens, or the peg of the axis (C2) vertebra.

**Oedema**[1] Edema.[2]

**OPG** aka Orthopantomogram, OPT, Panoramic view. A tomographic device specifically designed to demonstrate the mandible and part of the maxilla.

**Osgood-Schlatter's disease** aka Osgood-Schlatter lesion.

**Ossification** The process by which bone is formed. Most commonly bone forms from cartilage (e.g. a long bone); less commonly bone forms from membrane (e.g. skull). Ossification can also occur in the soft tissues either as the result of haemorrhage following trauma or due to chronic inflammation.

**Osteochondral fracture** A fracture involving a joint surface in which the fracture fragment consists of a small piece of bone and cartilage. The cartilaginous component is invisible on the plain radiograph. Example: an osteochondral fracture of the dome of the talus.

**PA** Postero-anterior. Indicates the direction of the x-ray beam as it passes through the patient.

**Paediatrics**[1] Pediatrics.[2]

**Palmar** Relating to the palm of the hand (i.e. the ventral surface).

**Paralytic ileus** aka Adynamic ileus.

**Paraspinal line** aka Paravertebral stripe. A vertical radiographic interface (or line) between the thoracic vertebrae and the adjacent lung seen on a frontal radiograph. This line is normally only seen on the left side of the thoracic vertebral bodies. The line is composed of the visceral and parietal pleura as they wrap around the sides of the vertebrae. Any process that displaces the pleura away from a vertebra may cause localized widening or bulging of a paraspinal line on either the left or the right side. In the context of trauma bulging or widening is usually due to a haematoma from a vertebral fracture.

**Periosteal new bone formation** aka Periosteal reaction, subperiosteal new bone formation. The appearance of a thin white line along part of the shaft of a long bone which appears to be separated from the cortex by a small space. The periosteum is invisible on a radiograph, and the reaction (or new bone) is a layer of ossification deep to the invisible periosteum. The small space between the white line and the bone is due to elevation of the periosteum by blood, pus, or tumour. In the context of trauma a periosteal reaction is a normal healing response.

**Plastic bowing fracture** aka Bowing fracture. A type of long bone fracture which occurs in children. A series of microfractures causes the bone to bend with no obvious abnormality of the cortex. Occurs most commonly in the forearm bones.

**Position (radiographic)** See: View.

**Projection (radiographic)** See: View.

**Pulled elbow**[1] aka Nursemaid's elbow.[2]

**Radiographer**[1] aka Radiographic technician[2] or Radiologic technologist.[2]

**Radionuclide investigation** See: Isotope investigation.

**Renal colic** aka Ureteral colic, Ureteric colic.

**Rolando fracture** **Y, V,** or **T** shaped intra-articular fracture of the base of the first metacarpal. A comminuted Bennett's fracture-dislocation. Invariably unstable.

**Rotation/rotational deformity** This is present when a fracture fragment has rotated on its long axis. Rotation is either external or internal (see illustration). Though rotation is most often / more readily diagnosed on clinical examination, it will sometimes be detectable from the radiograph. A rotational deformity will not correct itself spontaneously and surgical intervention is usually required. All fractures need to be evaluated in terms of position (see Table 1.2, pages 8-9); all long bone fractures should be checked to see if there is any suggestion of rotation.

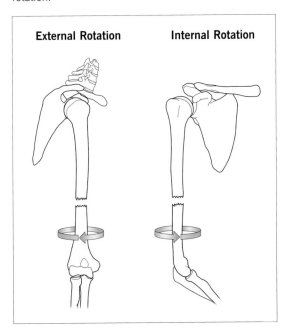

External Rotation     Internal Rotation

**RTA**[1]  aka Road traffic accident[1], Motor vehicle accident (MVA).[2]

**Salter-Harris fracture**  aka Epiphyseal fracture. The Salter-Harris classification describes the radiographic appearance of the fractures which involve the epiphyseal plate. The classification has a particular relevance to prognosis.

**Scaphoid bone**[1]  aka Carpal navicular.[2]

**Scintigraphy**  See: Isotope investigation.

**Sclerotic**  Denotes a dense (white) line or area on a radiograph. This may be at the periphery or cortex of a bone (e.g. the sclerotic appearance of maturing callus surrounding a healing fracture), or traversing the shaft of a bone (e.g. an impacted fracture).

**Scrapper's fracture**[1]  aka Fighter's fracture. See: Boxer's fracture.

**Screening**[1]  aka Fluoroscopy[1, 2,] Fluoroscopic screening. See: Fluoroscopy.

**Skier's thumb**  aka Gamekeeper's thumb. Rupture or stretching of the ulnar collateral ligament at the first carpo-metacarpal joint. See: Gamekeeper's thumb.

**Skyline view**  aka Sunrise or Sunset view. A tangential radiograph of the knee which provides a supero-inferior view of the patella and the patello-femoral joint.

**Snuff box**  aka Anatomical snuff box. The area on the radial side of the carpus formed where the extensor tendons of the thumb pass over the base of the first metacarpal. Tenderness at this site is frequently associated with a scaphoid fracture or a fracture of the styloid process of the radius.

**Spinal canal**  aka Vertebral canal. The space surrounded by the bone ring formed by the vertebral body anteriorly, the pedicles laterally and the lamina posterolaterally.

**Stress fracture**  aka Fatigue fracture, March fracture. A fracture resulting from minor but repeated injury.

**Subluxation**  The articular surface of one bone maintains some contact with the articular surface of the adjacent bone. The joint surfaces are no longer congruous but contact has not been completely disrupted.

**Sudeck's atrophy**  aka Reflex sympathetic dystrophy syndrome. Severe localised reduction in bone density. Most commonly occurs as a result of trauma with or without a fracture.

**Sustentaculum tali**  A medially projecting shelf of bone arising from the calcaneum. The upper surface of this shelf forms an articular surface for the medial part of the talus.

**Suture**  A junction between adjacent membranous bones in the skull which is separated by a narrow layer of fibrous tissue. See also: Accessory suture.

**Suture diastasis** aka Spread suture. Abnormal widening or separation of a skull suture.

**Swimmer's view** A lateral radiographic projection used to show the cervico-thoracic junction. The name derives from the patient's position: one arm is fully extended whilst the other remains by the side. The position simulates that of a swimmer doing either the back stroke or the crawl (freestyle).

**SXR** Skull radiograph.

**Symphysis** A joint between adjacent bones lined by hyaline cartilage and stabilised by fibrocartilage and ligaments. Example: symphysis pubis.

**Synchondrosis** The site of a persistent plate of cartilage between adjacent bones, at which little or no movement occurs. Example: zygomatico-frontal synchondrosis.

**Technician[2]** aka Radiographer[1], Radiographic Technician[2], Radiologic Technologist[2].

**Terry Thomas sign** Widening of the scapho-lunate joint usually consequent on a ligamentous injury. Named after a 20th century British comedian and actor whose trademark feature was to smile broadly and show an unusually wide gap between the upper incisors. See: the Madonna[1, 2] sign.

**Tibial plafond** The distal articular surface of the tibia.

**TMJ** Tempero-mandibular joint.

**Torus** Used to describe a type of long bone fracture seen in children. The cortex is buckled or wrinkled. Derived from the description of a particular shape of architectural moulding.

**Towne's view** Skull radiograph obtained with the x-ray beam angled so as to show the occipital bone clear of the overlying facial bones.

**Trapezium bone[1]** aka Greater multangular.[2]

**Trapezoid bone[1]** aka Lesser multangular.[2]

**Triquetral bone** aka Triquetrum.

**Tuberosity** Any prominence on a bone to which a tendon or tendons are attached (e.g. tuberosity of the base of the fifth metatarsal).

**Valgus** An angular deformity at a joint or fracture site in which the distal bone (or bone fragment) is deviated away from the midline.

**Varus** An angular deformity at a joint or fracture site in which the deviation of the distal bone (or bone fragment) is towards the midline.

**Ventral** Relating to the anterior (flexor) aspect of the body or body part (e.g. a limb). See: Dorsal.

**Vertical beam radiograph**  Denotes the orientation of the x-ray beam with respect to the floor. The beam is at right angles to the floor.

**View**  aka Projection, Position, or Method. In the context of diagnostic radiology this refers to the position of the patient or of the x-ray tube when a radiographic exposure occurs. Examples: frontal view, lateral view.

**Volar**  Relating to the palm of the hand or the sole of the foot.

**Well corticated**  A term used to describe the appearance of the periphery of a bone (e.g. an accessory ossicle) where it is seen to have a dense smooth margin. This appearance contrasts with the incompletely corticated margin of a fracture fragment.

**Wormian bone or bones**  A small bone in the skull occurring within a suture. Most frequently in the lambdoid suture. These bones are present in many normal infants up to the age of one year. They may be single or multiple.

# INDEX